MY UNREMARKABLE BRAIN

MY UNREMARKABLE BRAIN

A FAT-FUELED ADVENTURE INTO THE WORLD OF EPILEPSY AND THE KETOGENIC DIET

DAVID MOORE ROBINSON

NDP

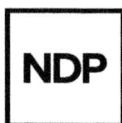

NEW DEGREE PRESS

MY UNREMARKABLE BRAIN
*A Fat-Fueled Adventure into the World of
Epilepsy and the Ketogenic Diet*

ISBN   978-1-63676-536-5 *Paperback*
        978-1-63676-083-4 *Kindle Ebook*
        978-1-63676-084-1 *Ebook*

for Judy, my muse

TABLE OF CONTENTS

———

INTRODUCTION

In all fairness, it was two days before Christmas—Christmas Eve-Eve, I guess you'd say. Still a workday for most of us, but it's also a day when coworkers are somehow nowhere to be found, and whoever's left has trouble even finding their desk beneath the pile of cookies and candies, let alone getting any work done. In short, it was the perfect day to get my head examined.

I mean that literally. After ten years of peace and quiet, my long-dormant epilepsy had been acting up and my doctor had ordered an EEG and an MRI, brain scans that might give some clue about what I've got going on between my ears.

I have done this before, I reminded myself, *and I've made it through.* The pilled hospital robe, the darkened room...all strange and familiar. The task was simple enough: lie on this thin foam mattress and hold completely still while the machine slides you in and out of this coffin-sized machine. I did my best to calm my quickening breath, ignore my itching nose, and generally keep from freaking out.

Somehow or other, the time did pass, and apparently the chunky, baby-blue-scrubs-clad radiologist got whatever pictures he needed from behind the protection of the inch-thick window. "That's it," he said.

I sat up as he came back into the room. "How does it look?" I asked.

"Well," he shrugged, "you have a brain." I'm not 100 percent sure, but I seem to remember he was eating a cookie at the time. I shot him a look, and he gave his real answer, the one he tells all the patients before he sends them on their way: "Your doctor will call you in a couple of days with the results."

***

Like I said, it was a Friday and a holiday weekend, so I didn't really expect to hear from the doctor right away. But in the end, I never heard from him at all. The weekend came and went, the holiday week came and went, the new year arrived, and still no word from the doctor, but one day an envelope showed up in the mail from the radiology center. Assuming it was a bill, I slid my finger in the corner of the envelope and readied myself for a long session of haggling with the insurance company.

When I opened it, though, I was surprised to find it was not a bill. It was the actual MRI report itself. I read through it—if you can call what I did reading. As an English major with zero medical background, I read this report the way a kindergartner might read Dostoyevsky. "Procedure...Findings..."

I recognized some of the letters and numbers, but I had no idea what they represented.

What I did understand, though, was the "impression," also known as the final conclusion at the bottom of the page. The conclusion read: "Normal MRI of an unremarkable brain."

Sounds about right, I thought. Almost reassuring, in a way, to have confirmed in black and white with medical annotation what my elementary school teachers had always told me. I decided "unremarkable," in this context, is good, in the same upside-down medical way a "negative" cancer screening is a positive thing in life. I shoved the report in a desk drawer and tried not to think about it.

It's a powerful thing, though, seeing pictures of your own brain. Standing alone in the living room, puzzling over a report intended for professional eyes only...that experience ignited something in me. I wanted to know more—to figure something out for myself. I wanted to take charge of my own brain.

***

In one way, I had been on this trajectory for a while. As a middle-aged "fathlete" with a healthy dose of vanity, I'd been searching for years for the best way to eat, drink, sleep, and live to perform the best I could in workouts and to lose the spare tire gradually being inflated on my midsection.

I spent hours poring over books, reading articles, watching videos, and listening to experts. One thing led to another, and I began to discover there might just be a connection between my desire for good physical health and my need for better neurological health.

We are—each of us—owners, users, and sole proprietors of one human brain and one human body. Billions of neurons. Trillions of cells. A massive corporation with ourself as CEO. Isn't it incumbent on us to learn all we can about this organization? To find the best way to run it? That's what this book is about.

My experience with the radiology lab sent me on a search for the ways to take care of my body and my brain. What I discovered along the way was surprising and counterintuitive. I learned many of the myths serving as health truths (such as fruit smoothies are super-foods or cholesterol is a deadly poison) are a recipe for health disaster. I learned weight management is not a matter of simple calorie math, and I learned food might be the best medicine for a whole range of diseases, from diabetes to Alzheimer's—to even my own epilepsy.

***

This matters. We are living in an age in which 60 percent of Americans suffer from chronic disease.[1] Sick is the new normal. How did we get here? And how do we get out of here?

Through my own journey as a middle-aged guy with epilepsy, I've learned it's on us to find the lifestyle that brings us

---

1   "Chronic Diseases in America," Centers for Disease Control and Prevention, last modified September 24, 2020.

health and happiness. I've discovered principles anyone can use, whatever your situation, to thrive and live your best life. This book is about taking responsibility for your own health.

As you join me on my own journey, my hope is my experience will challenge and inspire you to go out and make your own path. We are stronger than we know. It's time to harness our strength, step up, and live large—no matter what life throws your way. If I, with my unremarkable brain, can figure it out, then so can you.

HOW NOT TO READ
THIS BOOK

———

This is not a how-to book, it's not a guidebook, and it's most certainly not a medical advice book. I'm not a doctor—rather far from it. I'm just an English major with a curiosity about diet, health, fitness, and (by necessity) epilepsy.

This book is many things: a story about a science experiment, told from the point of view of the subject; a travelogue of a crazy ride into a world of where fad meets science, and community converges around the shared experience of empowerment; a series of insights gleaned from interviews with some of the most innovative and iconoclastic researchers, practitioners, thinkers, and writers in the world of health today. My hope is in sharing these stories, I might entertain you, inspire you, and encourage you to think about whether it might be possible to advocate for and improve your own health, wherever you may be in life right now.

Even as I write this, COVID-19 (nastiest yet of all the COVIDs) is running roughshod over the earth. Doctors, researchers, and English majors alike struggle to understand the disease—its causes, its effects, its prevention, and its outcome. Meanwhile, in the vacuum of good information, armchair experts are a font of bizarre ideas, and sincere and frightened citizens are doing everything from mega-dosing vitamins to injecting themselves with Clorox.

In the midst of this environment, writing a book about unconventional and sometimes controversial health interventions runs the risk of being fraught at best and irresponsible at worst. I will take pains to clarify where I stray from the path of medical orthodoxy, but I also ask you to use your own critical eye and best judgment.

***

This book is divided into three sections. In the first, I tell the story of how this onetime college athlete went from being a "tall guy" to being a "big guy," my subsequent journey into the crazy world of American diet culture, and how I found, in the low-carbohydrate diet, an approach that works for me.

The second section focuses on my discovery of the connection between diet and brain health—not only for people like myself who live with epilepsy, but for all sorts of other people—and the fascinating and still-emerging science behind the diet-brain connection.

In the third and final section, I bring together lessons I've learned from interviewing dozens of leaders in the low-carb community, including researchers, physicians, patients, entrepreneurs, journalists, and more. I'll share the wisdom I've gained over the years of this journey and some principles you can apply to find your own path to health and wellness.

The ketogenic diet, which this book explores in some detail, is a medically approved therapy for epilepsy. A current list of physicians and other professionals who administer this diet can be found on The Charlie Foundation's website (www.charliefoundation.org), and there's a directory of low-carb-friendly doctors on www.lowcarbusa.org. Please (for the love of God, man, *please!*) consult with one of them, or with your own doctor, before undertaking any dietary or lifestyle changes.

Thanks, and enjoy the ride!

David Robinson
October 20, 2020

PART ONE

THE FAT-FUELED BODY

CHAPTER 1

FROM ATHLETE TO "FATHLETE"

———

I still remember the exact moment when I became an athlete.

It was an ordinary fall afternoon, gray and damp, and I'd showed up once again at the big concrete garage serving as a boathouse for my college rowing team's daily workout. Our coach had scheduled an erg test for the day's workout.

Now, there are fewer phrases that strike more fear into the quivering heart of a young rower than "erg test." The Concept II Rowing Ergometer, or erg, is a gray, nondescript piece of fitness equipment using the simple mechanisms of a sliding seat, wooden handle, bicycle chain, and fan to inflict torture on the user. The motion of sliding back and forth and pulling the handle against the resistance of the fan mimics the action of rowing in the boat. Coaches everywhere—from middle school teams to Olympic teams—use this same machine to test the fitness of their rowers.

As a gangly, shy eighteen-year-old, I'd had a tough time adjusting to college life. So, when a girl in the student commons shoved a flyer in my hand and suggested I go out for crew, I was floored. "You'd be awesome," she said.

Awesome? Me? I'd never been *awesome* at much of anything—certainly nothing athletic. I'd never quite grown into my body and getting my hands or feet to be in the right place just when the ball was arriving or getting my muscles to fire in the order needed to properly throw or kick was more of an effort of organization than I could ever seem to master. A good day in gym class was one in which I was picked second-to-last, instead of last. To me, sports meant smelly equipment, nonsensical rules, and mostly a lot of embarrassment.

But I showed up for rowing practice that week and I found, to my surprise, it wasn't a blush-inducing shame-fest in the same way other sports were. In college, the first year of crew is called the "novice" year, and indeed, that word choice was my saving grace. Just like in any other sport, I had no idea what I was doing, but here *no one* knew what they were doing. It was terrific.

***

Our coach was the opposite of any gym coach I'd ever had. A tall, soft-spoken man with a grey goatee, he was part teacher, part guru: the perfect coach for a shy kid who wasn't sure he belonged. We'd had several erg tests by this particular day, so I knew what was expected: pull on the handle as hard and fast as you can as many times as you can until the little display thingy says five thousand meters. Coach made it clear on these periodic erg tests we were to do our best, but he didn't apply the pressure of a high-stakes assessment. It was just a check-in to see our progress.

But on that day, I was worried. I was struggling outside of rowing—in classes, with missing home—with all the stuff making up the freshman experience. On this particular day, I'd gotten back a math test and I wasn't happy about the score, and I'd stayed up late working on a paper the night before. In fact, I'd begun to wonder whether rowing, and whether college at all, was for me. In today's parlance, I just wasn't feeling it.

Ten ergs lined up side-by-side along the length of the boathouse, and ten of us boys took our perches and began to warm up. Coach walked down the line, making some notes on his clipboard.

"I don't know, Coach," I said as he wrote my name, "I'm not having a great day today." I don't know what I expected—maybe pity, or a pep talk, or to be excused from practice. Whatever it was, I didn't get it.

"Well," said Coach, "this is where you turn it into a good day."

I understood what he meant: your excuses are no good here. Do the work, and the result will speak for itself. I shook off my lethargy, gathered my strength, and when he called "Ready-all, row," I attacked the machine, pouring all of my negativity and anxiety into the handle with every stroke.

I don't remember the time I pulled that day, but I remember it was a personal best. I remember I broke some barrier I'd been bumping against up to that point. Most of all, I remember Coach's words when he came around to scribble my time on his clipboard: "I knew you had it in you."

That incident has stuck with me for all these years because of the lesson it taught me. An erg test—a check-in, a test of fitness, a gauge of progress—was not just a reflection of my fitness, nor of my overall state in life. It was a chance to *alter* my state in life. Taking on this challenge, giving it my all, and succeeding provided me the power to turn things around and would have ripple effects on my studies, my relationships, and my happiness. The same can be said of any challenge: a race, a game, a workout, or a big project in school or at the office. When we refuse to shrink from the challenge, we make our lives bigger. This is the power of athletics.

That was the moment when I turned into a college athlete. I continued to row throughout my four years. I devoted half of my waking hours and all of my energy to a sport that offered no scholarships, no status, and no accolades—nothing much more than sidelong looks from my classmates who wondered about those oddballs who wake up at five o'clock every morning. I felt at home in the boat. It became my identity—both a rower and a student, often in that order. Rowing was my home base during college. Paradoxically, spending time on the water—skimming across it backward by digging into it with an oar blade—was grounding for me. The water was where, again and again, I could turn bad days into good days. No matter how much I gave, rowing gave back much more.

***

Twenty years later, it is my thirty-ninth birthday. I'm at a long table in an Italian restaurant in Boston with my wife Judy, my mother, and a dozen of my best friends. But it's not my birthday that's brought us together.

The third weekend in October in Boston means only one thing: The Head of the Charles—part-rowing regatta, part-rowing convention, and part-city-wide party, The Charles is the biggest event of the year for American rowers. That it happens to be my birthday is a happy coincidence. It's my first year with the Alexandria Community Rowing club, and my first year back in the boat since college.

So, what happened? That was the question that came to me every time I caught a surprise glimpse of my reflection in a window or a mirror. That familiar smack of disappointment, which I buried as quickly as I could, was usually washed down by a snack or a beer. Over the course of fifteen years, my love-hate relationship with physical activity had swung back to the other pole way too often, and usually stuck there.

In the decade and a half since college, I'd moved five times— Philadelphia, New York, Colorado, Miami, DC—and it seemed like each move had taken me further from the water and further from my glory days. As I approached forty years old, my exercise consisted of walking the dog around the block and running out to the store for a six-pack of IPA.

Like every good thing in my life, it was my wife who brought athletics back to me. We had just moved to Alexandria,

Virginia, and she was working from home, which meant all she had for company was me and our dog Jake. In other words, she was starving for some intelligent conversation.

She learned about a local running group called the Ladies' B&RB. "B&RB" was her coach's invention; it stood for "Beginners and Re-Beginners." I still love this name with its implicit acknowledgment that health and fitness are journeys with lots of ups and downs and starts and re-starts.

She began with one- and two-mile runs, eventually working her way up to running half-marathons. Because I'm an amazing husband (and because it often involved a trip to someplace cool), I'd accompany her, jogging to different points on the course to take action photos of her and her friends— pink-faced, chatting, and laughing through the miles. Her "running buddies," as they called one other, became her peer group and her best friends.

I wanted in. I missed the active life—the kinship, the camaraderie, the body I didn't have to hide under supposedly "slimming" black t-shirts. I started picking up the pace on my walks with Jake, extending the distance here and there.

It wasn't easy at first. My affinity for IPAs and my grad-school smoking hobby turned my body into a rusty machine. To steal a phrase from John "The Penguin" Bingham in his book *The Accidental Athlete*, I'd spent years treating my body like it was disposable. Add to this the fact that the DC area is one of the fittest in the country, and my nice, quiet runs along the river usually left me a panting, red-faced pile of shame.[2]

***

One day I was running (okay, plodding) along the river, and I happened upon a big, blue building labeled "Dee Campbell Boathouse." I wondered...could this be a rowing club?

For a long time, I hesitated. DC is filled with young, type-A go-getters who run triathlons before power breakfasts and lift weights during their power lunches. There was no way my nearly-forty-year-old body would do anything but embarrass me. But I finally got around to doing some googling and making some phone calls and was invited down to see the place by Alan, the head of membership for the masters' program.

The next morning, I peeled myself out of bed at five o'clock and met Alan at the boathouse door. He was tall, lean, kindly, and several years my senior. He was dressed in rowing shorts and a t-shirt, as he'd already been working out for a good half an hour. "Welcome," he said, in a pleasant British accent. "Let me show you about." The boathouse was a huge, cavernous garage with three large bays housing dozens of racing shells. In the upstairs area, thirty ergs were arranged neatly in rows, and a handful of people worked at them or at the weight benches and other equipment.

---

2   Michael Rodio, "Washington, DC, is America's Fittest City for 2016." *Men's Journal,* accessed October 22, 2020.

It did my heart good hearing once again the high, familiar whine of half a dozen flywheels running in synch. Contrary to my expectation, the guys and gals at the club were of all ages, all shapes, and all sizes. In fact, it looked like I'd be on the younger side of the men's group. It was November, and Alan explained the club had a winter conditioning program starting after Thanksgiving.

Perfect, I thought. I could get in shape and lose some of this beer belly before the season started, and thereby minimize my embarrassment in the boat.

From across the room came a short, muscular man with silvering hair and a broad smile. "Rich," he said, extending his hand.

Alan introduced me as a "prospective member." "Dave might join us for winter conditioning next month," Alan said.

"Big Dave!" Rich grinned. "Why not join now? No time like the present!"

And that was it. I was in—no longer a prospective member, just a member. And with a new nickname, at that. I jumped into winter conditioning with all I had. Monday, Wednesday, and Friday mornings—come hell or high-hangover—I forced myself to get my butt down there and go through the paces of the grueling workouts Jaime, the women's coach, seemed to invent on the fly. Did I end up red-faced, sweating like a pig, and struggling to keep up? Sure, and I loved every minute of it. On the erg, my muscles found the old groove—legs, back, arms; arms, back, legs—and I felt home again.

Winter conditioning gave way to on-the-water rowing season, and I quickly found a home in the sixth seat of the eight-man boat. We were a ragtag bunch of guys, and we didn't win a whole lot of races, but we quickly became close. There's something about spending every morning together suffering, pouring yourself into the task of pulling on an oar over and over again, synchronizing your efforts with eight others, and ignoring the sheer folly of heading out again and again, only wind up an hour later at exactly the same dock where you began. Something about it brings people together.

By the time my thirty-ninth birthday came the following fall, Alan, Rich, Bill, Ed, JJ, and the rest of my rowing buddies had become my closest friends. Daniel Brown captures the effect beautifully in *The Boys in the Boat*: "What mattered more than how hard a man rowed was how well everything he did in the boat harmonized with what the other fellows were doing. And a man couldn't harmonize with his crewmates unless he opened his heart to them. He had to care about his crew."[3]

People think I'm crazy disciplined (or perhaps just crazy) to wake up early on a weekday to go work out. But in truth, when my alarm goes off at 4:48 a.m. I hop out of the bed and head straight out the door—no snooze and no hesitation. Why? Because I know, after going out on the water and getting a good sweat on, I'll hit Starbucks with my boys, where we'll spend a few minutes talking and cracking jokes before heading to work. I call this my "Blue Zone time," named after

---

3   Daniel James Brown, *The Boys in the Boat: Nine Americans and their Epic Quest for Gold at the 1936 Berlin Olympics* (New York: Viking, 2013).

the well-known book by Dan Buettner that shows social connectedness is associated with a longer lifespan. There's more and more research showing such post-workout socialization can lead to better performance, health, and longevity.[4]

For years, I fell into the trap so many Americans do, equating "exercise" with "working out" alone at a soulless gym. It was a boring and solitary experience I, for some strange reason, was never able to stick with for very long. Now exercise is a major part of my life.

There's research showing my experience is not unique. Kelly McGonigal, Stanford University professor of psychology and aerobics class teacher, in her book *The Joy of Movement* says, "Physical activity influences many other brain chemicals, including those that give you energy, alleviate worry, and help you bond with others. It reduces inflammation in the brain, which over time can protect against depression, anxiety, and loneliness." She shows how exercise also "remodels the physical structure of your brain to make you more receptive to joy and social connection."[5]

Do I row as fast as I used to? Not by a long shot. Have I achieved perfect, Adonis-like proportions? Please. These days I'm more what you might call a "fathlete" than an athlete. I can't even claim to have anywhere near perfect attendance at practice every day. But in rowing I've learned to

---

4 "Exercising and Socializing Can Lead to Better Mental Health," November 7, 2013, in *Health in a Heartbeat*, produced by UF Health Podcasts, podcast, MP3 audio, 1:59.

5 Kelly McGonigal, *The Joy of Movement* (New York: Penguin Random House, 2019), Introduction, Kindle.

get over myself, to get past some of these hang-ups, to have fun in moving my body, and, most importantly, to begin and re-begin.

CHAPTER 2

CHUNKY AS I WANNA BE

———

I spent the better part of my twenties teaching high school in New York City. It was a stressful, difficult, exhausting job, and I loved it. Kids in the Bronx had a unique perspective— an energy and a love of life at odds with the worn, gritty, industrial surroundings of city.

It was an active job. I was on my feet all day teaching, then I stayed after school to coach a small but not-particularly-talented group of boys in track and field. Lunch was a sleeve of potato wedges and a burrito from the hybrid KFC/Taco Bell across the street, scarfed down between grading papers and griping with colleagues, or sometimes just a banana and a coffee at the corner bodega. Dinner was forkfuls of takeout with my roommates in between nodding to sleep on the couch.

I lasted five years—longer than most of my colleagues—but eventually I burned out, or wore out perhaps. Although I loved the wild roller coaster of a day spent rushing to-and-fro in overcrowded hallways, talking and screaming and circus-clowning my way through life fifty minutes at a time, my brain did not. It was during this time I had my first seizure. I still wonder whether the stress of life is what caused the circuits in my brain to finally overload.

***

In part because of that development, I decided it was now or never if I wanted to go back to school for a degree in creative writing, and in no time at all I exchanged the concrete canyons of New York for the actual canyons of Colorado. Bleary-eyed subway rides became quiet mornings sipping coffee and scribbling in a dream journal. Matching wits with hyperactive teens all day became languid afternoons reading on the couch.

It's no wonder I got fat. My new anti-seizure medication may have played a part, but such a dramatic shift in lifestyle without much of a change in my eating (there was still a Taco Bell across the street from my apartment) certainly can't be ignored. I turned thirty in my first year of graduate school. The pounds gathered around my middle with determination and ferocity. Friends and relatives came to visit and barely recognized me. Judy, my long-distance girlfriend at the time, poked my stomach and said, tactfully, "You're gonna work on this, right?"

At the end of the year, I went back to visit my old school. I was out of place, wearing a pair of baggy jeans and polo I'd bought at the thrift store (being a student now, it was hard to keep up with my need for ever-larger clothing) instead of the khakis, button-down, and tie I'd been required to wear as a teacher.

I strolled the halls, chatting with old colleagues and saying happy hellos all around. I was talking with our school secretary when Janae, a girl I'd taught the year before, came around the corner. She stopped, taken aback, when she finally recognized me. Peering at me above the wire rim of her eyeglasses, she blurted out, "Mister! You're as chunky as you wanna be!"

***

I finished school three years older and sixty pounds heavier than I started. I still remember the look of horror on poor Judy's face when at our wedding—a month after graduation—I joked to my brothers, "Now that I'm married, I can *really* let myself go."

I tried not to. Instead, I became a serial dieter. Usually it would work like this: I'd find a new diet or program and get all excited about it, read the book, buy the materials, throw myself in, commit really hard for a while, stumble, get frustrated, give up, and then find something else. Here's a little sampling of the diets I've tried, in no particular order:

The Fat Smash Diet
The Biggest Loser Diet
The Three Season Diet
Weight Watchers (twice)
SparkPeople
MyFitnessPal
FitBit (not a diet, I know, but let's throw it in for good measure)
The Wild Diet
The Primal Diet

The Abs Diet
The Calorie Myth
The Fast Metabolism Diet
Clean Eating
Total Body Transformation
The Shape of Your Life
I Can Make You Slim
The Gabriel Method
Never Binge Again
Full-Filled

These are just the ones I remember off the top of my head. As unmanly as it is to say, yes, I've read diet books, and yes, I've been on diet programs—ad nauseam. The fact is, the diet-industrial complex is so vast, and there's so much conflicting information out there, you could spend a lifetime sweating on a treadmill of nonsense. I found it useful to develop a sort of taxonomy of diets to help make some sense of it all. Some categories might be:

Celebrity Diets: These are the books written by (or more likely, ghostwritten for) some movie, television, or internet celebrity whose smiling, healthy, well-lit face appears on the cover. The implicit message is if you want to look like a red-carpeter, this diet will get you there. One example would be Laird Hamilton's online exercise and fitness program. (Yes, at one point I actually believed looking like a Hawaiian lifelong surfing champion was as simple as drinking "superfood coffee" and doing a couple of lat pulldowns.) Let's also throw in *The Biggest Loser* diet and the *Outside Magazine* diet which trade in on the popularity of a particular TV show, publication, or pop culture phenomenon.

Mental Diets: It's all in your head, according to these diets. If only you knew how to control yourself, think good thoughts, and groove to a positive vibe, then your weight would normalize effortlessly and easily. These include self-hypnosis programs, meditations, self-discipline tricks, and the like. (Of course, if it doesn't work, you must not be thinking hard enough. You might have to sign up for one-on-one therapy—for hundreds of dollars a session—to really get the results you want.)

"I-Lost-Weight-and-So-Can-You" Diets: There are a ton of these out there. In science, an experiment where N=1 is not worth much of anything. But in the publishing world, a set of rock-hard abs and the anecdotal evidence of, "Hey, I ate nothing but sprouted-grain muesli for a month, and the results speak for themselves" is usually enough to get someone a book contract.

Programs: You can be sure you're following a diet when they say, "It's not a diet, it's a lifestyle!" In programs, the lifestyle is one of monthly bills. These are the folks who have figured out it's better to sell you a subscription than a book, often knowing full well you'll start, quit, then restart again many times over a multi-year period. (Here's to you, Oprah!)[6]

Mythology Diets: These are based on the idea that sometime in the misty past (like, when we were all cavemen), or in some far-off and exotic land (say, Crete or Okinawa), people had it all figured out. All you have to do is eat the way they did,

6   Traci Mann, "Oprah's Investment in Weight Watchers Was Smart Because the Program Doesn't Work," *Brow Beat* (blog), *Slate*, November 3, 2015.

or the way we think they probably did, at any rate. I'll also throw in here the many "back to nature" diets that tell you to cut out any stench of modernity from your day-to-day life, get in tune with the living world, and stop harming fellow creatures—the kind of feel-good stuff that makes organic markets the fastest growing industry in all of food-dom.[7]

I'm sure there are more. As I say, I've fallen for lots of gimmicks, and as they say, the bigger you are, the harder you fall. That's not to say these are all bad, though. Each have at least a nugget or two of valuable information to offer. Each has taught me something, and I'm sure each of them works for someone. But every time I found myself navigating a labyrinthine set of rules, activities, and do's and don'ts, I'd know on some level trying to complicate my eating habits would eventually fall apart.

That's why it was so refreshing when my dietary wanderings eventually let me to a book called *Fitness Confidential*.

TAKING "DIETS" OUT OF MY DIET

"Your good intentions have been stolen, and I'm here to help you get them back!" This is the catchphrase of author Vinnie Tortorich, veteran fitness trainer and renegade podcaster. In his bestselling book, he reflects on thirty years working as a Hollywood trainer, and in chapters like "Why Calories In, Calories Out is Bullshit," and "Use the Gym, Don't Let it Use You," he blows the lid off the myths, ruses, and hustles

---

7   "Organic Market Overview," USDA Economic Research Service, United States Department of Agriculture, last modified September 10, 2020.

perpetuated upon the well-meaning public by those who promise weight loss and beach-worthy abs.[8]

"No one wakes up saying, 'I want to be four hundred pounds today.' People want to do the right thing, but they've been given the wrong information" by food manufacturers, government lobbyists, and the media.[9]

It's a message that resonates; over the past nine years, the podcast has garnered over a million downloads a month and a loyal, almost rabid following, including a Facebook group of nearly thirty thousand members. Along the way, Tortorich has gone on to start Pure Vitamin Club, Pure Coffee Club, and NSNG Foods, as well as produce a film called *Fat: A Documentary* which rocketed to number one on iTunes, beating out *Free Solo* to become the top-rated documentary of all time, before going on to do the same thing on Amazon. (If the name rings a bell, you may have seen it on one of the many airline flights on which it's been featured entertainment.)

His book *Fitness Confidential,* didn't fit into any of my categories, really. Part-memoir, part-manifesto, it was the strangest health and fitness book I'd ever read. But I liked it. Tortorich's dietary advice, given offhandedly somewhere in the middle of the book, consisted of only four letters: "NSNG." No Sugar, No Grains.

---

8   Vinnie Tortorich with Dean Lorey, *Fitness Confidential*, performed by Vinnie Tortorich (Los Angeles: Pistachio Press, 2013), Audiobook.

9   Vinnie Tortorich and Andy Schreiber, "Throwback: On the Road, Young and Obese," October 12, 2015 in *Fitness Confidential,* produced by Vinnie Tortorich, podcast, MP3 audio, 6:01.

I had been poking around the neighborhood of low-carb diets for some time. "Paleo" sounded kind of silly; after all, as my friend Rich likes to say, if a caveman found a doughnut lying on the ground, he'd eat it. "Low-carb" sounded too restrictive. My sister would say, "of course you're going to lose weight if you cut out a third of all food." But NSNG sounded simple—too simple, really. But here was this guy who claimed since the 1980s, it's been the plan he's used with everyone from Hollywood starlets to get them red-carpet ready to average people looking to lose lots of weight.

In interviewing Tortorich for this book, I asked him about the importance of NSNG to him personally. He believes not only has it kept him healthy, it's kept him alive.

In addition to being a trainer for others, Tortorich spent his life as a top-level athlete. He played Division-1 football in college and later became an elite-level distance athlete, competing in races like the Furnace Creek 508—a torturous, nonstop, five-hundred-plus-mile cycling race through Death Valley, the hottest place on earth.

One day in 2007 while training, he got some bad news. "I had gone to my doctor to get a red-blood-cell test, as part of my training," he said. "She called me on my cell phone that Saturday. She's a friend of mine, but still it was unusual for her to call me on Saturday because she knew I was on my long training ride. 'Don't ride another foot,' she said. 'Get into a cab and get down here immediately.'"

The diagnosis was not good: leukemia. Still salty with sweat from his ride, he asked the doctor what stage he was in. Stage three? Stage four? "You're beyond stages," she said. It was at such an advanced state, she said, 80 percent of his bone marrow was cancerous. "I couldn't believe it," he said. "Here I was coming straight off an all-day ride, and someone is telling me I'm about to die."

Immediately, he had to park the bike, cancel all of his clients, and dedicate himself full-time to fighting the cancer. "I don't like to say I beat cancer," he told me. "The chemo and the cancer were fighting it out, and my body was the arena." He survived, beating the odds, and after months of torturous treatment, his oncologist pronounced him cancer-free.

"At the time, I lived in Hollywood—the land of fruits and nuts—and everybody and their brother came to me and said, 'Hey man, you need to start smoking pot, you need to get onto the vegan diet, you need to eat beets everyday...'" he laughed.

"I'll never forget the day my friend said, 'Oh yeah, eight ounces of wheatgrass a day. One time, years earlier, I had tried to drink *one* ounce of wheatgrass. I had heartburn the rest of the day. All I could do was burp up this horrible grass taste, like I ate out of a lawnmower or something. I couldn't imagine having *two* ounces, much less *eight* ounces.'"

So, at his appointment with his oncologist, a research doctor at Cedar Sinai, he ran it by her. "I said, 'Doc, everyone's telling me to eat a macro diet, a micro diet, all these other things. Is there anything to any of this?'"

"She said, 'Aren't you the guy who tells your clients to avoid sugar and grains? Well, do that.'"

"I said, 'Really?'"

"She said, 'Yeah. No one's really talking about it, but there's some research coming out that cancer feeds on sugar.'"

Ever since that one, offhand comment, Tortorich has lived a strict low-carb lifestyle, and for twelve years he's remained cancer-free. "The kind of cancer I have, hairy cell leukemia, never really goes away. There's always a small amount in the body. My doctor told me I'd probably be back on chemo before long—about four years, on average. She said if you go all the way to five years, you're really doing great." That was twelve years ago, and Tortorich has been off sugar—and stayed off the chemo—ever since.

***

It's hard to reconcile the seriousness of Tortorich's personal story with the sheer silliness of his podcast. Every episode, he and his cohost Anna Vocino would bust the myths of the latest nonsense fitness crazes, from cool-sculpting, to juice-cleansing, to "v-steaming" (in which women apply steam to their nether regions for some reason).[10]

I found myself laughing uncontrollably—a welcome break from my commute—and nodding along with Tortorich's outrage at the sheer lunacy of health advice today. His personal take on dieting—no sugars, no grains—seemed brilliant in its simplicity. Forget about counting, tracking, weighing,

---

10   Vinnie Tortorich and Anna Vocino, "Listener Questions," February 9, 2015 in *Fitness Confidential*, produced by Vinnie Tortorich, podcast, MP3 audio, 8:45.

measuring, checking the phases of the moon...just cut out those two things. But I still wondered: as entertaining as he was, could this guy really know what he was talking about?

CHAPTER 3

THE LAND OF THE LOW-CARB LUMINARIES

———

By the time he reached the age of sixty-five, William was fed up. At five-and-a-half feet tall, he tipped the scales at a hefty two-hundred-and-two pounds, putting his BMI around thirty-three—well within the range of what is generally considered obese.

He was an active guy—a skilled carpenter with a thriving business as an undertaker—and was finding his weight was getting in the way of his lifestyle. On the advice of a doctor, he'd tried rowing but found, much to his frustration, exercise only made him feel hungrier.

He called his excess fat a "parasite," an "insidious, creeping enemy" stealing away his life and his happiness. He avoided crowded places. He endured the sneers and comments of his friends and acquaintances. "I could not stoop to tie my shoe," he lamented.[11]

But it wasn't his frustrations with his weight which led him to see Dr. William Harvey. Rather, it was a mysterious episode of hearing loss. Dr. Harvey was an ear, nose, and throat specialist, but William's weight was an interesting puzzle to Dr. Harvey, who had recently been studying the liver and its role in diabetes.

At one lecture, Harvey heard the crazy idea that maybe what a person eats had something to do with the development of diabetes and obesity. So, when two-hundred-plus-pound William waddled in, Dr. Harvey wrote an unusual prescription: William should "abstain as much as possible" from bread, butter, sugar, beer, and potatoes, which William admitted "had been the main (and I thought innocent) elements of my existence." Dr. Harvey advised he swap these foods out for meat, fish, poultry, vegetables, and fruit, and trade the beer for tea without sugar or "a good claret."[12]

Within five months, William lost nearly fifty pounds, and became not just a convert, but a writer about and zealous promoter of his new way of eating, dedicating much of his own time and money "to the benefit of suffering humanity."[13]

***

---

11 William Banting, "Letter on Corpulence, Addressed to the Public," Internet Archive, accessed October 22, 2020.

12 Ibid.

13 Ibid.

There are several remarkable things about William's story: his frustration and sadness over years of failed attempts at weight loss, his rapid and easy success once he cut out starches and sweets, and his chance encounter with an ear, nose and throat doctor. Also remarkable is the fact this unorthodox diet goes against the current USDA recommendations, and a doctor could actually get in trouble for prescribing it. But perhaps the most remarkable fact of all is this happened way back in the year 1862.

William Banting is often considered the "father" of the low-carb diet. Having discovered Dr. Harvey's magic cure for obesity, he wrote an article about it and sent it around to several medical journals. When this failed, he self-published the pamphlet "Letter on Corpulence, Addressed to the Public," which quickly became a bestseller, selling over sixty-three thousand copies in the UK alone through the remainder of the decade. (At one point, his last name "banting" became a household verb, meaning "to go on a weight-loss diet.")[14]

Banting's story resonated with me. Like him, I had felt the sting of "remarks and sneers, frequently painful in society, and which, even on the strongest mind, have an unhappy tendency." Like him, I'd tried exercise—including rowing—and found little help. Like him, I had no idea low-fat foods like bread and potatoes were major contributors to my weight (though I had a pretty good idea the beer wasn't helping).

---

14   Gary Taubes, *Why We Get Fat: And What to Do About It*, (New York: Alfred A. Knopf, 2011), 153.

The story is one of many mind-blowing tales in Gary Taubes's book *Why We Get Fat (And What to do About it)*, which challenges conventional wisdom about diet and weight loss. In the first chapter alone, Taubes pulls more than a dozen examples from the fields of anthropology and public health of populations described as *both* malnourished and obese. These studies span the globe and more than fifty years, and time and again hardworking, impoverished populations suffer the dual problems of being under-nourished and overweight.[15]

One incredibly vexing story is drawn from a 2005 article by Benjamin Caballero, head of human nutrition at Johns Hopkins University. Caballero's article describes the slums of Brazil as filled with "thin, stunted young children, exhibiting the typical signs of undernutrition," but the surprising fact that at the same time, "their mothers were generally overweight."[16] How to explain this phenomenon?

Taubes says examples like these challenge our ideas of weight gain as a simple result of eating too much: "If we believe that these mothers were overweight because they ate too much, and we know the children are thin and stunted because they're not getting enough food, then we're assuming that the mothers were consuming superfluous calories that they could have given to their children to allow them to thrive. In other words, the mothers are willing to starve their children so that they themselves can overeat. This goes against everything we know about maternal behavior."[17]

---

15   Ibid, 24-32.

16   Ibid.

17   Ibid.

Stories like this help to prove Taubes's overall point: it's not just the *number* of calories we eat, it's the *type* of calories that matter.

One of the biggest paradigmatic shifts I learned from Taubes was to begin thinking of weight as a matter of biology rather than morality. We see obesity as the "wages" for the dual sins of gluttony and sloth.[18] All it takes to lose weight, we are told, is to eat less and move more. If you're heavy, then it means you've failed this simple task and given in to your base, heathen urges. That spare tire of yours? It's the scarlet letter you deserve for being unable to control yourself (and thus, fat-shaming is completely justified).

The surprising thing is it wasn't always this way. Taubes has spent a lot of time diving deep into the history of weight loss and has unearthed some remarkable stories, including this one:

In the first part of the twentieth century, Germany was the epicenter of scientific research—so much so American college students majoring in science were often required to learn the German language so they could keep up with the latest findings. At the time, there was general agreement among scientists that obesity was a disease primarily of hormone dysregulation, and a lot of German research was focused on discovering exactly which hormones were out of whack in the overweight person.

---

18   Susan Perry, "Carbs, Not Fats (Nor Gluttony, Nor Sloth) Are What's Making Us Fat, Says Author of Controversial New Book," *MinnPost*, January 26, 2011.

So, when did all that change? Well, some really, really bad stuff went down in Germany, so after World War II, all German research was lost or ignored. At around the same time, and for about the same reasons, researchers became more interested in the problem of starvation than that of obesity. In the aftermath of the war, there were lots of people around the world who either had starved or were still starving, and the calorie was a useful way of thinking about food's ability to provide energy and sustenance.[19]

***

The problem is, we never matured beyond the simple notion of "calories in, calories out." This idea is not false, Taubes says, it's just simplistic.[20] Imagine you're asking, "Why is the airport so crowded?" and the only answer you get is, "Because there are more people coming in than leaving." You'd say, "Okay, but why are none of the planes leaving?" Maybe there's bad weather. Maybe the workers are striking. Maybe a renegade tribe of sheep is refusing to clear the runway. The answer to this second question, not the first, holds the key to getting the airport cleared out.

Taubes's book outlines several possible answers to the second question, and most revolve around how our hormones, not our willpower or moral fortitude, regulate how many calories we store versus how many we use for energy.[21] The science

---

19   Gary Taubes, "Obesity's 'No There There' Problem: A History of Causal Thinking in the Science," PowerPoint presentation, Low Carb USA Virtual San Diego 2020, August 29, 2020.

20   Taubes, *Why We Get Fat*, 74-75.

21   Ibid., 112-133.

is still ongoing, and the jury is still out on the exact causes and solutions. But maybe in the meantime we can at least let old Hester Prynne take off that big, red "F."

***

This was the real value of the *Fitness Confidential* podcast. In one of his five weekly shows, Tortorich interviewed a "luminary" in the field of health and fitness. Gary Taubes was the first of these I heard, and reading his book convinced me NSNG was worth a shot. Week after week, I discovered a whole world of thinkers and writers who were writing books about diet which weren't "diet books." They were books with covers not featuring a glossy, smiling photo of the author, illustrations of exercises, or weekly meal-plan grids. Instead, these volumes contained footnotes, appendices, and references...just like real books! Each one turned my world just a little bit more on its axis until, to quote another of Tortorich's favorite sayings, I "could not unsee" the truth I had learned and yearned for a chance to share it with everyone I knew.

CHAPTER 4

OF HYBRIDS, HUNGER, AND HUMAN BIOLOGY

So how is it cutting carbs leads to weight loss? Is it, as my sister said, the calorie reduction that necessarily comes from cutting out one-third of all food intake? Or is there something else at play? Here's an overview of science, given by a guy who barely passed high-school chemistry.

GETTING SAD

A favorite acronym for dietary gurus today is SAD, which stands for the Standard American Diet. It's a nice catchphrase, and a bit of a zinger, but it begs the question: what do Americans actually eat? Depending on who you listen to, we eat way too much red meat, too much fast food, too-large portions, too few fruits and veggies, too many snacks, too much sugar, too much caffeine...the list goes on and on.

If we zoom out to the macro level (specifically, the macro-nutrient level), the average American gets approximately:

- 50 percent of their calories from carbohydrates,
- 35 percent of their calories from fats, and
- 15 percent of their calories from protein.[22]

It's worth noting here these numbers are well within the US Dietary Guidelines, which tell us to eat:

- 45–65 percent of our calories from carbs,
- 25–35 percent of our calories from fats, and
- 10–30 percent of our calories from protein[23]

...even though it's the very same diet which has made 70 percent of us overweight or obese.[24] So yes, like good little children we are eating what we're told, and it's not working out for us.

Percentages are well and good, but what does this diet look like in real life? Let's start with the classic example of "fattening food:" Mickey D's. According to the McDonald's Nutrition Calculator website, a meal consisting of a Quarter Pounder, medium Coke, and medium fries contains:

- 141 grams of carbohydrates
- 40 grams of fats, and

---

22 Allen R. Last and Stephen A. Wilson, "Low-Carbohydrate Diets," *American Family Physician* 73, no. 11 (June 2006); 1942-1948.

23 "Appendix 7. Nutritional Goals for Age-Sex Groups Based on Dietary Reference Intakes and Dietary Guidelines Recommendations," Office of Disease Prevention and Health Promotion, accessed October 22, 2020.

24 "Obesity and Overweight," FastStats—Overweight Prevalence, Centers for Disease Control and Prevention, last modified February 28, 2020.

- 35 grams of protein.[25]

If we do a little math, and use the USDA's guidelines on number of calories per gram of each macronutrient, we end up with:

- 564 calories of carbs, or 53 percent,
- 360 calories of fat, or 34 percent, and
- 140 calories of protein, or 13 percent.[26]

In other words, a McDonald's meal—something most people would agree represents a really "unhealthy" choice—represents the typical meal for the typical American. And, oh yeah, it is exactly what we're "supposed" to be eating. I'm no math-a-magician, but something here isn't adding up.

EAT LESS, MOVE MORE

So, okay. To go on a low-carb diet is to simply eat half as much food, right? Half as many calories in, same calories out...boom: weight loss! Easy, right?

Not so fast. Cutting your intake in half may work in the short term, but it's not going to last. That experiment has been done in the form of a TV show called *The Biggest Loser*. Remember this one? Producers spent sixteen weeks fat-shaming contestants by dressing them up in silly helmets and dangling

---

25   "Nutrition Calculator," McDonalds, accessed October 22, 2020.

26   "How Many Calories are in One Gram of Fat, Carbohydrate, or Protein?" USDA National Agricultural Library, Food and Nutrition Information Center, accessed October 22, 2020.

them from ropes while trainers yelled at them. You know...
for fitness.

Well, a recent study followed up with the contestants years
after. Researchers found six years after the show, thirteen out
of fourteen former losers had regained most of the weight
they'd lost. What's more, their metabolic rate—the number
of calories the body burns at rest—had dropped by an average of 607 calories a day, as compared to before the show.[27]
This means if they now eat the same number of calories after
the show as they had before the show (a familiar phenomenon to any of us who've gone on a diet and then reverted to
our old ways), they would gain more weight now than they
had before.

In other words, starving yourself thin will eventually back-
fire on you.

The Biggest Loser experiment shows the failure of the calorie in/calorie out theory of weight loss, also known as the
"energy balance" theory. This theory is based on a principle
from physics known as the first law of thermodynamics. This
law states that in a closed system, energy can neither be created nor destroyed, meaning calories coming into the body
(say, a quarter pounder meal) must be either burned for fuel
(to keep you warm, to take a walk, or to use your brain) or
stored somewhere (like around your waist).

---

27 "6 Years after *The Biggest Loser*, Metabolism is Slower and Weight is Back
Up," *Scientific American*, May 11, 2016.

Gary Taubes acknowledges the essential truth of this theory, but then asks, "Yes, but so what? ...Thermodynamics tells us that if we get fatter and heavier, more energy enters our body than leaves it. Overeating means we're consuming more energy than we're expending. It says the same thing in a different way. Neither happens to answer the question why."[28]

Answering the question *why*, Taubes argues, requires an understanding not of physics, but of biology. Quoting a 1998 report by the National Institute of Health, Taubes writes, understanding the "why" requires "the integration of social, behavioral, cultural, physiological metabolic and genetic factors."[29] His two books *Good Calories, Bad Calories* and *Why We Get Fat and What to Do About It* explore these various factors in great detail. But for a clear understanding of one of the most important factors, I turned to Dr. Jason Fung.

IT'S ALL ABOUT THE INSULIN, BABY

"I can make you fat," says Dr. Fung. "Actually, I can make anybody fat. How? By prescribing insulin. It won't matter that you have willpower, or that you exercise. It won't matter what you choose to eat. You will get fat. It's simply a matter of enough insulin and enough time."[30]

Dr. Fung's book *The Obesity Code* is an engaging, readable overview of the ways in which the calorie theory falls short

---

28 Gary Taubes, *Why We Get Fat*, 75-76.

29 Ibid.

30 Jason Fung, *The Obesity Code: Unlocking the Secrets of Weight Loss*, read by Brian Nishii, (Vancouver, BC: Greystone Books, 2016), Audible audio ed. 10 hrs, 9 min.

and how hormones play a central role in weight gain. As a nephrologist (kidney doctor), he has seen firsthand the sky-rocketing rates of obesity and diabetes in North America and has a unique understanding of the science behind it. Dr. Fung calls excess calories the "proximate" or immediate cause of obesity but not the "ultimate" cause.

"After puberty," Dr. Fung points out, "women on average carry close to 50 percent more body fat than men. This change occurs despite the fact that men consume more cal-ories than women. But why is this true?"[31] To understand the underlying cause, he says, we have to get beyond the "eat less, move more" conventional wisdom and look at how different foods function in the body.

In short, the foods we eat cause hormonal reactions. "In your body, nothing happens by accident. Every single physiologic process is a tight orchestration of hormonal signals. Whether our heart beats faster or slower is tightly controlled by hor-mones. Whether we urinate a lot or a little is tightly con-trolled by hormones. Whether the calories we eat are burned as energy or stored as body fat is also tightly controlled by hormones. So, the main problem of obesity is not necessarily the calories we eat, but how they are spent, and the main hormone we need to know about is insulin."

---

31   Ibid.

Insulin, Dr. Fung explains, is a "fat-storing hormone."[32] Its role in the body is to get glucose (a.k.a. sugar) out of the bloodstream. Here's how it goes:

1. You eat something—a steak, a doughnut, or whatever.
2. Your digestive system converts the carbohydrates in the food into glucose, which is released into the bloodstream.
3. Insulin is secreted by the pancreas. It escorts glucose into the cells of your body—the muscles, the organs, and other places where it's used for energy.
4. Leftover glucose is sent to the adipose tissue, where it's converted to fat and stored for later.

This is, of course, a way-oversimplified explanation, but it will work for now.

Over the weeks, months, and years, eating too many carbohydrates too often will raise insulin levels higher and higher. This is what happens in people with type two diabetes, whose cells become "deaf" to the effect of insulin. People with diabetes have high insulin levels all the time but also high blood sugar. The traditional solution is to inject more insulin, in order to clear the sugar out of the blood (where it can cause tissue damage). But as Dr. Fung shows from the research as well as his own clinical experience, this inevitably leads to increased fat storage.[33]

---

32 Jason Fung, "My Single Best Weight-Loss Tip," Diet Doctor, November 4, 2018.

33 Ibid.

In other words, insulin is a one-way street. It pushes calories into the fat cells and doesn't let them come back out. To lose body fat, then, you first need to lower insulin. This is where the low-carb diet comes into play.

YOUR BODY IS A HYBRID

Carbohydrates aren't the only thing you can burn for energy. There's another source of energy in the food you eat and in the rolls around your belt: fat.

My friend Michael drives a Prius, and when my license was suspended for having a seizure, he was kind enough give me a lift to work every day. On his car's dashboard, there's a little light showing how much electricity the car is using and how much gas. When the car is moving slowly down the block or cruising at highway speeds, it uses mostly electricity. Electricity is a nice, efficient, steady-burning fuel for the car.

But as a hybrid, the car also has a gasoline engine. When you step on the gas pedal to accelerate at a green light or to merge into fast-moving highway traffic, the car knows it has to recruit the gasoline engine to give it a quick blast of power and speed.

Your body is the same way. When you're at rest or exercising at an easy pace, most of your energy comes from fat. Let's say you're walking the dog—stop to sniff here and there, check your phone, etc. About 85 percent of your energy to do these things comes from fat.[34]

But let's say you're looking down at your phone thumbing out a quick text, and your dog catches sight of the mailman at the end of the block. He rips free of the leash and is tearing up the street before you know it. Your heart leaps and your legs spring into action, sprinting after the little bugger as fast as you can. For this kind of short-term, hard-core effort, the body switches over into sugar burning mode, calling on the limited supply of glucose stored in the muscles.

The body is designed this way, to switch easily between burning fat and burning glucose, ideally.

Elevated levels of insulin can mess with this system. In their comprehensive (and super science-y) book *The Art and Science of Low-Carbohydrate Performance*, researchers Jeff Volek and Stephen Phinney explain the use of fat for fuel "is principally controlled by the single hormone that *inhibits* its activity. That hormone is insulin. In other words, insulin is the primary gatekeeper of body fat. If your insulin levels are consistently high, fat usage is effectively blocked."[35]

In other words, it's like the electric motor of your Prius is busted. You have all this juice stored up in the big battery, but you're stuck driving gas station to gas station trying to get by on an inefficient motor.

---

34 Katarina Melzer, "Carbohydrate and Fat Utilization During Rest and Physical Activity," *Clinical Nutrition Espen* 6 no. 2 (Apri 2011): E45-E52.

35 Jeff S. Volek and Stephen D. Phinney, *The Art and Science of Low-Carbohydrate Performance* (New York: Beyond Obesity, 2012), 20, Kindle.

HANGRY?

How do you know if you've got a broken motor? There's one sure-fire sign, and it's become so common we even have a word for it: "hangry."

A combination of "hungry" and "angry," the word "hangry" was first coined in the fifties, but its use in the last few years (perhaps tellingly) has skyrocketed. Recent studies have validated hunger and mood swings do go hand-in-hand in many people, and the culprit is low blood sugar. When blood sugar begins to fall, "it triggers a cascade of hormones, including cortisol (a stress hormone) and adrenaline (the fight-or-flight hormone)."[36]

It looks like this:

1. On the way to work, you stop by Starbucks for a sugar-filled coffee flopaccino and a pastry.
2. The glucose from all of those carbs hit your bloodstream, giving you a shot of short-term energy.
3. Insulin does its thing, clearing out all the blood glucose and, at the same time, keeping you from dipping into your fat stores.
4. You go from high blood sugar to low blood sugar, and your brain notices this change. By noon, it's throwing a temper tantrum, trying to get some more freaking sugar in there already.[37]

---

36 "Is Being 'Hangry' Really a Thing—or Just an Excuse?" Cleveland Clinic Heath Essentials, December 24, 2018.

37 Tro Kalayjian and Brian Lenzkes, "Episode 110: Dr. Ben Bikman is Back!" June 1, 2020 in *Low Carb MD Podcast*, podcast, MP3 audio 1:03:54.

This is what some people call the "blood sugar rollercoaster." How do you fix it? Many experts suggest you avoid the lows by eating more often. Writing in *The Globe and Mail*, dietician Leslie Beck says, "it's critical to eat every two to three hours to prevent your blood glucose from falling too low" in order "to ensure glucose enters your bloodstream at a steady, even pace throughout the day."[38]

So...stick to using the gas motor, just hit the station more often. This is the advice we've been hearing for years. But what if there's another way? The low-carbohydrate diet takes the opposite approach. It says what if, instead of trying to keep blood glucose high (and therefore insulin high), what if we try to keep it low?

Vinnie Tortorich calls it "remapping the system." When you cut way down on the carbohydrates, you get off the sugar roller coaster. You replace the starches and sugars with protein and fat. In so doing, you "teach" your body to burn fat again by not allowing it to live on carbs.[39] Instead of spending your day pumping your blood with sugar over and over again, you keep it at a constant, low level. This keeps insulin low, which in turn allows your body to use the efficient, clean-burning fuel known as fat.

And once the body gets onto the fat-burning train, it can switch seamlessly from burning fat from food, to burning

---

38   Leslie Beck, "I Have Low Blood Sugar—What Should I Eat?" *The Globe and Mail*, May 30, 2012.

39   Vinnie Tortorich, *Fitness Confidential*, Ch 6.

fat from the body. This is one reason why studies have shown people eating low-carb diets feel report feeling less hunger.[40]

Lower insulin = increased fat burning. Increased fat burning = less hunger. Less hunger = less overeating.

∗∗∗

This brings us full circle back to our old friend, the calorie. The calorie is nothing more than a unit of energy. The bottom line is your body's going to get the energy it needs from somewhere. If you feed it carbohydrates, it will get the energy from carbohydrates. If you feed it fat, it will get the energy from fat. Though some of my low-carb friends will probably skewer me for saying this, changing *what* you eat doesn't mean you can completely forget about *how much* you eat.

Low-carb eating isn't magic. It isn't a "hall pass" for weary dieters. It's simply a way to ease the transition from burning food to burning body fat by getting your body in the habit of burning fat—rather than carbohydrates—as fuel. The big advantage here is fatty foods are more satisfying than carb-filled foods and don't cause the same hormonal chaos, so you don't find yourself getting hungry all the time, meaning fewer snacks and fewer chances to overeat. But if you tend to eat out of habit or boredom rather than hunger, then you might not see the losses you're hoping for.

---

40   Sharon M. Nickols-Richardson et al, "Perceived Hunger Is Lower and Weight Loss Is Greater in Overweight Premenopausal Women Consuming a Low-Carbohydrate/High-Protein vs High-Carbohydrate/Low-Fat Diet," *Journal of the American Dietetic Association* 105 no. 9 (September 2005): 1433-143.

It took me a while to learn this (and, in fact, I still have to relearn it from time to time). In the meantime, I kept listening to podcasts, reading books, and beginning and re-beginning my efforts. Then, an unusual guest on Tortorich's podcast took my diet adventure in a whole new direction.

PART TWO

THE FAT-FUELED BRAIN

CHAPTER 5

WORLDS COLLIDING

———

I've heard it said bad days make for good stories. Well, my best story happened June 28, 2017. I only wish I was there to experience it. Here's how my friends tell it:

My wife Judy is at home on a Sunday afternoon taking a bit of a nap. Her phone rings, which is odd because it's been on "do not disturb" mode. She sees the number is mine, so she answers.

"Hello?" she says.

"Hello, is this Judy Robinson?" The voice on the other end—deep and serious—isn't mine.

"Yes...who is this?"

"Are you the spouse of David Robinson?"

"Yes...who is this?"

"I'm calling from the sheriff's office in eastern Pennsylvania. Your husband's been in an accident."

"Oh my God! Is he okay?"

"He's been taken to the hospital here. The fire chief has taken your dog Jake home to his house. We need you to come here to get them."

I have been away camping for the weekend, and Judy knows I'm spending this particular Sunday afternoon driving back home. She had gotten a text from me at my last stop in Wilkes-Barre, just a little while ago, and everything seemed fine.

Now, Judy doesn't drive. (It's a long story.) Half-panicked, half-dazed, she casts her mind about for someone to call—someone who would drop everything to drive three hours on a Sunday afternoon to the middle of nowhere to go retrieve her injured husband. She calls the first people who come to mind: my best friends and rowing teammates Rich and Bill.

***

The way they tell it, Rich and his wife Patricia are out having drinks and charcuterie at their favorite restaurant. Bill and his wife Jane are enjoying cocktails. But Judy's instinct is right. Drinks are abandoned, a plan is formed, and soon the five of them are piled in a minivan and speeding out of the city on "Operation: Rescue Big Dave."

Bill drives. Rich, who has been robbed of his charcuterie, repeatedly begs to stop at each passing McDonald's. "Come on! He's fine; he's Big Dave! Anyway, what's five minutes gonna do?"

Judy's hands grow white with wringing. "We're not stopping," Bill says. "Judy's gotta get to her man." Along the way, Judy fills them in on my backstory, telling them what I've never had the guts to: I have epilepsy

***

I'd had my first seizure when I was twenty-eight. This is unusual—many people think of epilepsy as a kids' disease—but it's not unheard of. In fact, one in ten Americans will have a seizure at some point in their lifetime, and one in twenty-six will develop epilepsy, which is defined simply as having two or more unprovoked seizures.[41]

After my first seizure, I was prescribed medication, monitored closely then distantly, and sent on my way.

I turned thirty. I turned forty. Day piled upon day, framed by the familiar ritual of swallowing a pill when I first woke up and swallowing another before I slept. I didn't love the grogginess that sometimes came with the meds, and sometimes I felt as if I'd lost a step, cognitively, but it was a bargain I was willing to strike. To be able to drive a car, get married, hold a job, work and get promoted, buy a house—in other words, live the normal ups and downs everyone experiences—was more than a fair bargain.

---

41   "Seizure First Aid," Centers for Disease Control and Prevention, last modified September 30, 2020.

To say I'd almost forgotten about it would be an overstatement—you never forget epilepsy—but in the course of ten years successfully seizure-free, I had grown less vigilant.

Then came the music.

Every seizure is different, just as every person is different. Doctors have identified many different types of seizures, but even within these categories there is variation. Like many people with epilepsy, my own seizures begin with what's called an "aura," an unusual sensory experience not founded in reality. Some people begin seeing things—bright lights, tunnel vision, even cartoon characters dancing through the room. Some feel the earth move, like a roller coaster or a plane entering an air pocket. For me, it's music.

It's hard to describe. Have you ever had a tune stuck in your head, and you just can't get it out? It's like that, times ten. I can physically hear the notes of the song, even as I know it's coming from inside my head. The music always seems familiar, yet I can't put my finger on the song. I often get the idea if only I can name that tune, the seizure won't come. Along with the music comes a sense of panic: my pulse quickens, I begin to sweat, and I feel lightheaded. It's happened enough now I know what it means, and my thoughts follow a familiar line. "What is that song? Oh, God. Oh, no. Oh, please, God, no. Not here. Not now...What is that damned song?"

Then, nothing.

That's why, on that sunny Sunday afternoon in June when my car radio started playing two songs at once, I knew what was happening. It had been a long time, but I recognized the cues. I clicked off the radio, wanting it to be a freak moment with the FM signal. "God no," I thought. "Not here."

I punched the button for my hazard lights, slowed the car and pulled onto the shoulder. The easing down of the vehicle belied the panic inside. I steered with my left hand while my right searched frantically through my backpack for my medication, hoping I could pop a pill quick and ward it off.

That's the last clear memory I have from that day. From there, I have only flashes: the inside of the ambulance, where I regained just enough consciousness to realize what had happened and muttered a sad, "Oh, nooooooh;" the face of the EMT who rode with me to the hospital, reassuring me I'd be all right; spotting my own car through the rear window of the ambulance, as if seeing it from an out-of-body experience—sitting in tall grass, on a slope, at a twisted and disturbing angle; the face of Judy, and the faces of my friends behind her, as I blushed dazedly at the awareness I was wearing only a thin, pilled hospital gown.

Where do you go when you can't trust your own brain? It's a question that rang in my head in the days following that seizure. There were no strobe lights, no extreme temperatures, and no club drugs in darkened corners—nothing to blame but my own brain acting up, refusing to cooperate with the agenda I'd set for the day. I felt frustrated and powerless.

TWO ROADS CONVERGE

It had been a year or so since I discovered low-carb eating—a year of reading, researching, thinking, and experimenting. I sometimes say I'd been playing at low carb: sticking to it a while, losing ten pounds or so, slacking off and re-gaining, and then telling myself to get back on the ball, in the usual cyclical pattern. In other words, it was just another diet.

I would go back to Tortorich's show, along with the half-dozen other podcasts I now listened to regularly, for motivation as well as for information. Sometimes I'd get a nugget I hadn't heard before. (For example, it's actually a *bad* idea to snack between meals; even if your snacks are low in carbs, they'll raise your insulin enough it stops burning body fat in favor of digesting the new calories.) Then I'd try to implement it.

Then Tortorich had a guest who truly blew my mind, and it wasn't a doctor, researcher, or dietician. It was a movie producer.

Even if you haven't heard of Jim Abrahams, you probably know his work—*Airplane, The Naked Gun, Hot Shots*. If you're familiar at all with the canon of goofy comedy, you know Abrahams's movies. If you're a guy who grew up as a socially awkward teenager in the eighties and nineties, you know them line-for-line. So, I sat up and took more than a little notice when I heard Tortorich introduce one of the gods of goofball comedy on his little podcast.

But it wasn't his long and storied Hollywood career which brought him on Tortorich's podcast. He was there to tell the story of his son, Charlie.

Charlie was born in 1992. One day, when he was one year old, Jim was pushing Charlie in a swing, when he saw the child's head twitch to one side and his arm jerk suddenly up in the air. "At first, I didn't think much of it," Abrahams said, but he mentioned it to his wife Nancy later that day. She confirmed she'd seen Charlie do the same thing several times before.[42]

"That was the beginning," he said. They started seeing a neurologist, but in a very short time, the seizures began to increase in frequency and intensity. "He wound up having seizures in the arms of the chiefs of pediatric neurology at Boston Children's Hospital, Seattle Children's Hospital, UCLA, LA Children's Hospital..." Doctor after doctor prescribed drug after drug in a vain attempt to control Charlie's seizures. At one point he was on four different medications. Charlie even had what Jim called "a horrendous brain surgery," but to no avail. "We lost hope," he said. "We were basically told, 'There is no hope.'"

For parents, epilepsy is a particularly terrible disease. "It was devastating," he said. "It turns the whole family upside down." Sleepless nights, stress, worry, family events interrupted by trips to the emergency room...such is the life of the family of a child who is seizing up to twelve times a day.

---

42   Vinnie Tortorich, "Fighting Seizures with Jim Abrahams and Susan Masino," November 25, 2016, in *Fitness Confidential Podcast*, podcast, MP3 audio 1:45:02.

One day, after one of the many neurology visits, Jim stopped at a medical library, desperate to learn and hoping to find there some new stone to overturn in his search for help. In several old medical textbooks and publications, he happened upon a mention of something called the ketogenic diet.

"It was shocking to me, because what they all said was that about a third of the kids with epilepsy as bad as Charlie's who go on a ketogenic diet had their seizures go away. Another third were significantly improved, and for the last third it doesn't work. Different doctors from different hospitals in seven different decades used the identical treatment on a similar patient population and had virtually identical outcomes. And yet, all of these folks we had taken Charlie to see never mentioned a word about diet."

Abrahams called Dr. John M. Freeman, a pediatric neurologist at Johns Hopkins University in Baltimore. Freeman was America's foremost—and perhaps only—voice for the use of a ketogenic diet in the treatment of epilepsy. He worked with Millicent Kelly, a dietitian who had been perfecting the diet at Hopkins for fifty years and seen hundreds of kids cured.

Dr. Freeman told them that 50–70 percent of the cases which come through his doors and get put on the diet have success in reducing or eliminating seizures—a better rate of success than any drug on the market. They flew to Baltimore, where Dr. Freeman put Charlie on the diet right away, and within a month, he was seizure-free and was weaned off of all four medications.

"Charlie went from a prognosis of a lifetime of seizures and what they call 'progressive retardation,' to...we got our son back and he was happy again, and our family could go on with life."

Charlie began to grow and progress like any other kid, and after a few years on the diet, he was weaned off of it too, going back to a standard diet. His seizures didn't return. Now, Charlie is an adult and teaches school; he's living a successful life.

Jim and Nancy Abrahams became vocal advocates for ketogenic diet therapies for pediatric epilepsy and began the Charlie Foundation, which for twenty-five years has been the leading source of information and inspiration on diet and epilepsy. Abrahams found a second career in patient advocacy, and his passion is largely responsible for the growing popularity of the ketogenic diet. But there's still a ways to go. "Even today," he says, "only one-and-a-half out of every ten thousand patients who would benefit from this treatment ever learn about it."

I was riveted by this episode. To hear Abrahams speak so passionately about his experience was incredibly moving. He still chokes up and cries when he describes his travails as a parent and his frustration at the medical establishment for not offering this life-saving therapy to more patients. I found myself crying along, shaking my head, and pounding my fist.

Could it be this diet I was pursuing, basically for vanity reasons, was the way to get my brain and my life back on track? I needed to find out.

CHAPTER 6

THAT FUNNY THING MY BRAIN DOES

———

Growing up, my little brother was the standout one. He was the youngest, and by far the most energetic of my siblings, and he gave my parents a run for their money.

Around age five or six, he started going into "trances," as we called them. Instead of his usual, frantic, restless self, he'd become a statue—staring into the middle distance, silent and motionless. He might be in the middle of a sentence. "Today at school I was...." Pause for one second, two seconds, five seconds, and he'd finish "...drawing a picture of a car," as if no time had passed.

After several doctor's visits, my mother got a diagnosis of epilepsy. His "trances" were, in fact, absence seizures. His brain would misfire, in much the same way it would in someone who was having a full-fledged grand mal seizure, but without the physical manifestations.

As I remember it, his youth was a series of meds—Ritalin for the ADHD, Depakote for the seizures, other medications to deal with the side effects of those medications, and new medications when the previous medications stopped working... It was a constant source of worry and stress for my mother, and it was no picnic for him.

My own first seizure didn't happen until I was twenty-eight. I was living in New York, hanging out with my roommates one weekday evening, when I suddenly felt lightheaded and woozy. I stood up out of the easy chair where I was sitting... and that was it. Next thing I remember was seeing the inside of an ambulance, the EMT telling me I'd "given us quite a scare there."

Given my family history, doctors at the hospital put me on medication right away. Dilantin, it was called. I was to take 100 mg three times a day, or that's what it was supposed to be. What the intern actually wrote on the pad was 300 mg three times a day.

Over the next week, the medication left me a zombie during the day and took me to weird, technicolor dreamscapes at night. My mother had come down to the city to see me and to accompany me to my first follow-up appointment with a neurologist on the east side.

"*This* is what you've been taking?" the neurologist asked me, looking at the pill bottle, "For how long?"

Within minutes I was back at the hospital getting pumped full of IV fluids and getting my blood measured for toxicity because of that mistake.

***

Anti-seizure medications are hard. By definition, they mess with your brain chemistry. They also mess with your mood, your weight, your sleep, your energy, and pretty much every other aspect of your life. I've noticed I feel less creative when I'm on my medication (which is an issue for a creative writer).

But hey, to prevent another seizure, it's a tradeoff I'm willing to make. The weight gain, though, has always been a tough one. This is America, after all—land of the vain. My body went all funhouse mirror at the same time I started on anti-seizure meds. It was correlation, not causation, but I've always wondered about the connection.

Thing is, other than that, I've been able to pretty much live in denial all this time. Having seen the troubles my brother went through, I knew I didn't want that. So somehow in my mind, I was able to separate from it—to tell myself my epilepsy was somehow different.

***

It's interesting, the power of a diagnosis. You wake up feeling different, or maybe not when you wake up, but at some other point in your day—at work, or in the car, or playing pickup with your friends.

Something happens inside you that feels...wrong—off, somehow. It might be a pain of the shooting, stabbing, aching, yanking, or radiating variety. It might be lack of pain, or a lack of any feeling at all. It might be a gap between here and here, where feeling should be, but it's gone missing.

At this point, you make a decision. You ignore it in the hopes it will go away, turning out to be just one of those things, or you freak out, hoping against hope it's not a mortal blow. Or you make a mental note, thinking, "that's not right...I'll have to look into that." If the pain is too intense, you deal with it right away. If it's something able to be put off until later, you put it off.

At least, that's what I do. When it comes to illness, I'd say I've always had a bias toward inaction. I'm an inveterate procrastinator—at school, at work, on my taxes—and this procrastinating mindset applies most of all to my own body. Many people exclaim in wonder when they hear cliché stories of the guy who, after suffering chest pain for eight hours finally, reluctantly, at his wife's insistence, drives himself to the ER, only to find he's had a massive coronary. I hear that and think, "Yeah. Sounds about right."

So, I didn't go to the doctor after my first aura. I didn't even learn it was an aura until after a thorough cross-examination in a hospital bed—along with a three-day stay during which I had nothing to do but replay the previous months of my life over and over in my mind.

My first full-on seizure happened on an otherwise unremarkable Wednesday night. My roommates and I were chatting and swapping stories about our day, arguing over what to order for dinner. Then I felt it, like a flashback to my first childhood experience of learning the power of the ocean— the fear of being lifted off the sand by unseen hands, my feet losing their grip on the earth, floating backward, falling upward.

There, in the living room with my buddies, I felt the same severing of ties with gravity. At the same time, a tunnel closed around me. I heard everything in the room, and I knew I was hearing it but refracted, as if I were in a long tunnel or a deep well and the voices of my friends were bouncing off the walls before they reached my ears.

I stood, hoping to clear my head. That's the last thing I remember. Next thing I knew, I was in an ambulance and headed toward a diagnosis.

A diagnosis is a powerful thing. It's concrete. It's that rare thing we all search for in life: an answer. The thing that went wrong in your knee, your chest, your back? That pain, that kink, that owie? It's a question—an effect searching for its cause. Once we get the cause, the thinking goes, we can get rid of the pain. But what do we know? The body is a complex system, full of organs and muscles and guts and viscera. The pain could signal a malfunction in any one of these things. It would take a lifetime of study to pinpoint the exact cause of this problem. So, we turn to those who have, indeed, dedicated their lives to just this study. We go to the doctor.

The doctor gives us knowledge and expertise, but she also gives us language. She enables us to put words to what we're feeling, allows us to deal with it.

***

In my case, I didn't deal with epilepsy particularly well. I kept it close to my chest like a secret. Because I was one of the lucky ones—among the half of people with epilepsy whose seizures are well-managed with medication—for a long time, I could count in my head the number of folks who knew.[43] They included my family, my roommates from New York, and my close friends from grad school. The question is, why keep it to myself?

It turns out I'm not alone. Writing in the journal *Social Problems*, sociologists Joseph W. Schneider and Peter Conrad first coined the term "Epilepsy Closet" in 1980, as a way of describing the difficulty people with epilepsy have telling others about their condition.[44] More recently, psychologist Sallie Baxendale conducted a survey of twenty-one films released between 2000 and 2014 featuring a character with epilepsy or having a seizure during a pivotal scene. She found "Epilepsy continues to be associated with the supernatural in modern cinematic output. Demonic possession and epilepsy now share a similar cinematic lexicon," adding, "All

43   Niu Tian et al, "Active Epilepsy and Seizure Control in Adults—United States, 2013 and 2015" *Morbidity and Mortality Weekly Report* 67 no 15 (April 20, 2018): 437-442.

44   Joseph W. Schneider and Peter Conrad, "In the Closet with Illness: Epilepsy, Stigma Potential and Information Control," *Social Problems* 28 no. 1 (October 1980): 32–44.

too often, a character has epilepsy to maximize the unease of the audience with them; it is a device that is used to signal 'this character is not like you.'"[45]

Maybe the fear is justified. In his memoir *A Mind Unraveled*, Kurt Eichenwald describes in painful detail the very real discrimination people with epilepsy sometimes face. "A look at online message boards shows postings from women who were told they would be disowned if they married an epileptic boyfriend and others fired from jobs or shunned by friends after a seizure. Until 1956, eighteen states allowed for forced sterilization of epileptic people, and marrying them was illegal in seventeen; Missouri kept its marriage ban on the books until 1980."[46]

I know, I know. It's 2020. We're past all that. We have become much better these days at acknowledging our biases and not judging others based on such things. But at the very least, the person in the throes of a seizure is a person who has lost control of their faculties, and let's face it, American culture still has certain ideas about people who are sick. They are weak, and we don't like weakness. I'll admit as a man in America, I have many of those ideas bumping around in the dank basement of my own subconscious.

So yes, I have kept it hidden. For one thing, it's not exactly something that comes up in everyday conversation ("You know, speaking of partial-complex seizures..."). Since for me

45   Sallie Baxendale, "Epilepsy on the Silver Screen in the 21st Century," *Epilepsy & Behavior* 57 pt B (April 2016): 270-274.

46   Kurt Eichenwald, *A Mind Unraveled: A Memoir*, read by the author, New York: Random House Audio, 2018, Audible audio ed., Introduction.

a seizure is not a regular occurrence (as I say, I've gone as much as a whole decade seizure-free), it's easier to skip the topic completely than to get into "all that stuff."

But more than that, it's knowing—or at least fearing—this one thing, a glitch in my brain wiring, has the power to define me as a person in a way I'm not entirely comfortable with. There are many labels I accept with pride: husband, teacher, rower; and many others that I accept with some reluctance: white guy, big guy, middle-aged-guy, doofus. But the label of "epileptic" (or to be PC about it, "person with epilepsy") is one I resist. The label feels heavy and all-consuming in a way that is out of proportion with the small role the disease plays in my day-to-day existence.

Many people aren't so lucky. Epilepsy is for them a constant companion, staring at them every time they look in a mirror. I'm a lucky epileptic. Medication works. For the most part, it works. I take a pill and I'm fine. Really, I'm fine.

***

But I could never really escape it. I've heard it said having epilepsy is like having a stalker. You know he's out there, but you don't know where. He might be hiding behind the bushes just across the lawn, or he might be hanging from a tree in the yard, watching and waiting to pounce. Or he might be all the way across town having decided to take the day off.

One of the things that makes epilepsy so difficult—besides, you know, the convulsions, loss of consciousness, and injuries—is the not knowing. My seizure in Pennsylvania was easily explained (at least in my own mind). I was under a lot of stress and pushing my body and brain through a tough couple of days. I was not being smart about getting my rest or giving myself what I need.

Others, however, have come on completely unremarkable days. Six months after Operation: Rescue Big Dave, I seized again. This time, it was during a meeting at work. It was mid-afternoon. My boss was wrapping up an hour and a half of marching orders. My coworker made a joke, and everyone started laughing.

Once again, there was the lightheadedness, the confusion, and the paper-towel-roll-over-the-ear hearing. My heart started racing in my chest. "Shit," I thought. "Not here."

I knew what it was. I tried to breathe, tried to will my brain to stop it. I remember my coworker, sitting next to me, frowning with concern. "Are you alright?" she said. "It's hot in here." Which it was. She scooped a handful of ice cubes out of her big cup of water and handed them to me. *Ice*, I thought. *Why not? I've never tried that before.*

I've never properly thanked her for her kindness, so let me take a minute to do it here. It may not seem to add up to a whole lot—a handful of ice from an already-finished cup of water—but to me, her hand might have been reaching down from the lifeboat while I sunk amid the battering waves.

It doesn't matter that it didn't keep the seizure from happening. If ice cured seizures, we'd have kicked this condition long ago. What matters is the attempt—the moment of trying to help, even as I descended into epilepsy's dark and scary place inside my brain.

I later learned all of my colleagues jumped in to help as I fell convulsing on the floor. One, a trained nurse, took control of the situation right away. Another sacrificed her coat to form a pillow under my head. A third called an ambulance. My boss called my Judy at work...and more, probably, I don't even know about.

As much as it took me off guard, they were doubly surprised. I had been deep in the epilepsy closet, but within four excruciating minutes, I was out.

They were great, I must say. In the weeks following, each of them reached out to me with words of comfort and offers of help. "The main thing is there's a lot of people here who love you and care about you," said one. I've never forgotten it.

I began to think it was time to listen to Jim Abrahams and his Charlie Foundation, to see what this low-carb thing could offer my brain, not just my body.

CHAPTER 7

THE HUNDRED-YEAR-OLD FAD DIET

Note: There exist several excellent histories of the ketogenic diet, written by learned medical professionals. This is not one of them.[47]

***

By the time I encountered Jim Abrahams, I had heard the term "keto" kicking around for a while. Mostly, in the context of Crossfit types looking to get ripped and shredded—the same dudes who were into "paleo" not too long ago. My

---

47   For a more thoughtful look at this topic, check out the work of Dr. James Wheless ("History and Origin of the Ketogenic Diet," appearing in *Epilepsy and the Ketogenic Diet*, Stafstrom and Rho, ed.); Dr. John Freeman et al (*The Ketogenic Diet: A Treatment for Epilepsy* and *Looking Back, A Career in Child Neurology*); and Dr. Eric Kossoff et al (*The Ketogenic and Modified Atkins Diets, 6th Edition: Treatments for Epilepsy and Other Disorders*). I owe a massive debt to these authors and would like to acknowledge and thank them for their work, which formed the foundation for the brief, selective, and woefully insufficient summary here.

impression was keto was just one step further out on the diet spectrum: a new, more extreme way to eat, and guys love stuff that's "extreme."

That's why I hadn't paid it much attention. Even Vinnie Tortorich, when asked about it, said you don't need to be in ketosis to lose weight. He admitted he himself lived in ketosis because of his cancer, but didn't necessarily recommend it for everyone. This was confusing enough that I went ahead and ignored it. If I could cut out most sugar and most grains, I'd probably be fine.

Popular media supported this belief. Keto is regularly referred to as a "fad diet," sometimes even being called dangerous.[48] It sounded like something to stay away from.

What I didn't know is, far from being a new craze, the ketogenic diet is actually a very specific protocol used in medicine and studied in lab experiments for a hundred years, and in some ways, even longer.

EPILEPSY IN THE WAY-BACK MACHINE
If you've ever seen one of those old-time photos of logs being floated down a river, you have an idea what it's like at the Vatican Museum.

It was the third day of our Italian vacation, and Judy and I had been fairly gorging ourselves on great food and great

---

48 "Keto Diet: Expert Reviews," US News and World Report Health, 2020 Best Diets Rankings, accessed October 22, 2020.

art. In one of my rare flashes of foresight, I'd booked us a visit to the Vatican Museum, a massive, sprawling collection of several thousand years' worth of art and sculpture. The place is so popular you need to book your tickets ahead of time, and visitors are so clueless that the busy streets outside are filled with chattering hawkers selling overpriced and/or counterfeit "last minute" tickets.

Unfortunately, the museum inside was no less crowded than the streets outside. Official tour groups competed for floor space with masses of tourists and classes of bored high school students. Bouncing our way through the crowd and taking in the paintings lining the walls, the statues holding down the room, and the murals adorning the ceiling...it was a dizzying experience.

I like to think perhaps, if I hadn't been quite so lost, confused, or disoriented at the time—if I hadn't at that point been so overwhelmed with a kind of "masterpiece fatigue" brought on by the bombardment of my senses by great work after great work—I might have noticed and lingered a while before Raphael's *The Transfiguration of Christ*.

The painting, Raphael's last, is notable for many reasons: it was commissioned by Cardinal Giulio de' Medici (the future Pope Clement) in a sort of contest with Sebastiano del Piombo, another painter of the age. Raphael painted it entirely with his own hands, rather than shopping out any of the work to his assistants, as was standard at that time. It won the contest, and Raphael celebrated with a "wild debauch" which is said to have resulted in his death by fever, and in his sixteenth-century biography of the painter, Giorgio Vasari calls the painting "the most famous, the most beautiful, and most divine."[49]

The painting is celebrated for its innovative and beautiful use of light and dark, for the complexity of its composition, and for the beauty of its human figures.[50] But it's notable, too, because it refers back to among the first documented uses of ketosis as a treatment for epilepsy.

The painting takes as its subject two episodes from the gospel. In the upper, predominant image, Jesus is seen floating in the heavens, bright against a backdrop of clouds and flanked by the prophets Elijah and Moses. In the lower, darker half of the frame, a crowd gathers at the foot of Mount Tabor, but its attention is divided between Jesus in his glory and a shirtless young boy whose body is twisted, arm is flailing, and eyes are rolling upward.

Writing about the painting in the journal *Epilepsia*, Dieter Janz notes, "By synchronizing both scenes, Raphael demonstrated a significant correspondence between Christ and the epileptic boy, which reveals the epileptic seizure as a symbolic representation of a transcendent event...In the Gospels, the metamorphosis caused by the epileptic seizure is used as

49   "The Life of Raphael, by Giorgio Vasari, Introduced by Jill Burke—A Preview," Issu, last modified April 5, 2016.

50   "The Transfiguration—by Raphael," Raphael Paintings, accessed October 22, 2020.

a simile for Christ's transfiguration through suffering, death, and resurrection."[51]

In Mark's version of the story, Jesus descends from Mount Tabor to join the hubbub below. His disciples have been trying unsuccessfully to help a man whose son is possessed by a demon. "And wherever it seizes him," says the man, "it throws him down; he foams at the mouth, gnashes his teeth, and becomes rigid" (Mark 9:18). After casting the demon away, the disciples ask Jesus why they were unable to help the boy. He tells them, "This kind can come out by nothing but prayer and fasting."

HIPPOCRATES: LET FOOD BE THY MEDICINE

Jesus was not the first to connect fasting and epilepsy. Four hundred years earlier, a healer named Hippocrates took a less spiritual view of epilepsy treatment. Considered the father of medicine, Hippocrates sought to apply reason and science to the craft of healing the body.[52] In *The Sacred Disease*, he argues rather than "incantations" and rituals, it is "enforcing abstinence from baths and many articles of food which are unwholesome to men in diseases" which helps eliminate a patient's seizures.[53]

---

51 Deiter Janz, "Epilepsy, Viewed Metaphysically: An Interpretation of the Biblical Story of the Epileptic Boy and of Raphael's Transfiguration," *Epilepsia* 27 (August 1986): 316-322.

52 *Encyclopedia Britannica Online*, s.v. "Hippocrates: Greek Physician," accessed October 22, 2020.

53 "On the Sacred Disease by Hippocrates," MIT Internet Classics Archive, accessed October 22, 2020.

In fairness, Hippocrates advocated fasting for a whole lot of things—for everything from fever to mental illness. In fact, he called it the "physician within."[54]

HEALTH NUTS: BERNARR MACFADDEN AND HUGH CONKLIN

Nor was Hippocrates the only one who believed in the curative powers of fasting. Throughout the ages, the idea of purification and abstinence from food has been touted by everyone from healers, spiritual leaders, and shamans to health advocates. Somewhere in the middle of this spectrum could be placed one of the most colorful characters in this story, Bernarr Macfadden.

Macfadden was a fitness and health do-it-yourselfer. He was self-taught and self-appointed as a "Kinistherapist" and "Teacher of Higher Physical Culture" (titles he invented himself). He was even self-named, having changed his birthname Bernard to "Bernarr" (evocative, he hoped, of a lion's roar).

Credited as the father of bodybuilding (and by extension, godfather of the gym selfie), Macfadden's fifty-year career built an empire of fitness magazines (featuring, yes, gym selfies), natural-food restaurants, and "healthorium" retreat centers. He zealously promoted vigorous exercise along with a diet of vegetables and eggs, plus such interventions as

---

54 "Fasting and Purification: The Physician Within," Greek Medicine.Net, accessed October 22, 2020.

walking outside barefoot, sleeping on the floor, standing on one's head, and regular pulling of one's own hair.[55]

He also railed against the prevailing medical ideas of the day, believing people could live to one-hundred-and-twenty years of age if they lived cleanly and avoided medical treatment, eventually going so far as to develop "the conviction that the American Medical Association was trying to poison the wells on his country estate."[56]

Macfadden's healthorium was described by a visitor as a hotbed of unconventional ideas: "everybody [there] enjoyed a fad of his or her own. There was a little brown woman like the shriveled inside of an old walnut, who believed you should imbibe no fluid other than that found in the eating of fruits... There was a man from Philadelphia who ate nothing but raw meat. He had eruptions all over his body from the diet but still persisted in it. There were several young Italian naturefolk who ate nothing but vegetables and fruit, raw."

But Macfadden had many followers. His *Physical Culture* magazine had a circulation in the hundreds of thousands and converts to his philosophy included Upton Sinclair and Charles Atlas. At his healthorium in Battle Creek, Michigan, (where Macfadden was testing a milk cure for cancer while also waging battle with the competing sanitarium of cereal magnates C.W. Post and the Kellogg brothers) Macfadden found another follower in Dr. Hugh W. Conklin.

---

55 Ben Yagoda, "The True Story of Bernard Macfadden," *American Heritage*, December, 1981.

56 Ibid.

Conklin, a doctor of osteopathy, was particularly impressed by Macfadden's idea of fasting to "alleviate and cure about any disease, including asthma, bladder disease, diabetes, prostate disease, epilepsy, impotence, paralysis, liver and kidney disease, and eye troubles."[57]

Conklin applied Macfadden's fasting cure in his own practice, believing epilepsy had its origins in the intestines.[58] In a 1922 article by *The New York Times*, Conklin is quoted as saying after fasting for thirty days, many of his patients "are never afflicted by fits again." In children under eleven, he cured thirty-five out of thirty-seven cases, and "we effect cures in older patients from 50 to 60 percent of the cases we undertake."[59]

FROM FASTING TO FAT

Even before Conklin's article brought widespread attention to the treatment, other doctors had joined in using starvation to treat epilepsy. Dr. H. Rawle Geyelin, of the New York Presbyterian Hospital, began to use it in his own practice after Conklin treated a young cousin of his through several fasting periods and helping eliminate the child's seizures[60] Dr. Geyelin published his own results in 1921 on thirty-six patients, 87 percent of whom became seizure-free.

---

57 James W. Wheless, "History and Origin of the Ketogenic Diet," in *Epilepsy and the Ketogenic Diet*, ed. Carl E. Stafstrom and Jong Rho, MD (Totowa, NJ: Humana Press, 2004), 31–38.

58 Ibid.

59 "Fasting as Epilepsy Cure," *New York Times*, July 6, 1922.

60 Wheless, "History," 34.

Over the next ten years, several case reports were published in which fasting was shown to be at least partially effective for seizure reduction or elimination. Some patients became seizure-free only while fasting, while for others the seizures didn't return after they resumed eating.[61]

Why did it work? This was the question which intrigued Charles Howland, a wealthy New York lawyer whose son had become seizure-free in Dr. Conklin's care after all other treatments had failed. He funded studies by several doctors, including his brother Dr. John Howland of Johns Hopkins, Dr. Geyelin, and Dr. Stanley Cobb of Harvard. They found a clue in, of all places, pee.[62]

***

There weren't many things doctors could monitor in patients back then; they lacked the advanced medical equipment and thorough testing we have today. One thing they could measure, though, was urine. In studying patients whose seizures were well-controlled by fasting, Dr. Geyelin discovered their urine was measurably acidic. He reported this at the AMA convention in Boston. Dr. W. G. Lennox, a young cardiologist at the time, was "thrilled by Geyelin's demonstration" and joined Dr. Stanley Cobb in studying the problem.[63]

Lennox and Cobb studied the urine of a group of five patients (with Lennox himself serving as the control group) who were

---

61 Ibid.
62 Ibid.
63 Ibid.

put on various fasting and eating regimens. They found the uric acid lowered when the fast was broken with carbohydrates, but not when patients were fed 40 percent cream. "Simple absence of food or dearth of carbohydrate in the body forced the body to burn acid-forming fat," Lennox reported.[64]

Around the same time, Dr. Russell Wilder at the Mayo Clinic wrote, "Ketone bodies are formed from fat and protein whenever a disproportion exists between the amount of fatty acid and the amount of sugar," and "It is possible to provoke ketogenesis by feeding diets which are rich in fats and low in carbohydrates."[65] The ketogenic diet was born.

The next ten years saw a surge in publications on the ketogenic diet for epilepsy—discussing its effectiveness, protocols for its use, and particular formulations. Another Mayo Clinic pediatrist, Dr. M.G. Peterman, put the diet into use and published a standard formulation. He was the first to note improvements in behavior and cognitive performance that came along with the diet: "an increased interest and alertness...the children slept better and were more easily disciplined."[66]

Over the next twenty years, use of the diet spread to the point where, according to Dr. James Wheless, it appeared in "almost every comprehensive textbook on epilepsy in childhood that appeared between 1941 and 1980. Most of these

---

64 Ibid.

65 Eric Kossoff, MD et al, *The Ketogenic and Modified Atkins Diets: Treatments for Epilepsy and Other Disorders*, 6th ed. (New York: Demos Health, 2016), 43.

66 Wheless, "History," 39.

texts had full chapters describing the diet, telling how to initiate it and how to calculate meal plans."[67] In the 1960s, Dr. Lennox summarized the many studies over the preceding forty years by saying, "probably one-third of the children who maintain an adequate ketogenic diet for a prolonged period become seizure-free and another one-third are much improved."[68]

THE VANISHING DIET

So, what happened? How is it a treatment widely known to help a majority of patients just faded away? Why did the Abrahamses have to travel all the way across the country just to find a doctor who would administer the diet? In a word, drugs.

In 1937, phenytoin was discovered by doctors Tracy J. Putnam and H. Houston Merritt. It was found to be effective in controlling convulsions without the powerful sedative effects of the previous go-to drug, phenobarbital. The promise of new and more effective pharmaceutical cures drew researchers' and physicians' attention away from studying diet.[69] Diets, after all, are hard to stick to. They're expensive. They can be messy. How much easier and neater was it to simply prescribe a pill and send the patient on their way? Even if Dilantin had some pretty rough side effects (rashes, bone disease, lymphoma...) and even if was only effective somewhere between

---

67   Wheless, "History," 40.

68   William G. Lennox, *Epilepsy and Related Disorders* Vol 2: (Boston: Little, Brown and Company, 1960): 734-739, 824-832.

69   Kossoff et al, *The Ketogenic and Modified Atkins Diets*, 44.

27 and 70 percent of the time, it was okay because the great promise of pharmacology is that a new and better drug is always just about to be discovered.[70]

KEEPERS OF THE FLAME

The shift of researchers' focus to finding pharmaceutical solutions did yield results. There are now twenty different anti-epileptic drugs on the market which can be used to treat a wide variety of different types of seizures with pretty good effectiveness. A neurologist will prescribe one of these medications based on the type of seizures the patient is experiencing. Around 50 percent of the time, this works and the patient is seizure-free, or close to it.[71]

But what about everyone else? If the first drug doesn't work, the doctor will try another. This helps another 11 percent of patients. If this trial leads to an error, then a third drug is in order. But by that time the odds go way down; the third drug helps only another 2 percent of folks. In other words, the returns diminish the deeper you go into the drug roster. In the words of a recent, thirty-year study, "Despite the availability of many new AEDs with differing mechanisms of action, overall outcomes in newly diagnosed epilepsy have not improved...More than one-third of patients experience epilepsy that remains uncontrolled."[72]

---

70 "Phenytoin," Epilepsy Foundation, accessed October 22, 2020.

71 "Drug Resistant Epilepsy and New AEDs: Two Perspectives," *Epilepsy Currents* 18, no. 5 (September-October, 2018):

72 Ibid.

This is where the ketogenic diet comes in. It became—and is still used today as—a last resort for those unlucky patients whose seizures don't respond to medication. But it wouldn't be, if it weren't for a few key figures.

DR. SAMUEL LIVINGSTON

Dr. Samuel Livingston began at the Johns Hopkins Epilepsy Clinic in 1936. Writing in 1973, he remembered at the time the number of patients "whose seizures were controlled sufficiently to enable them to function normally was relatively small, approximately 10 percent."[73]

Over the next thirty-seven years, Livingston writes, that number rose steadily to 60 percent. Livingston credits many factors, including better diagnostic tools, newer drugs and procedures, and the ketogenic diet. "Improved technique in the administration of the ketogenic diet has also contributed to the better outlook for the child with epilepsy. This regimen is an excellent form of therapy for certain types of epileptic seizures in children." At the same time, he warns "specific factors such as the age of the patient, the type of epilepsy, and the ability of both patient and parents to cooperate satisfactorily, influence its effectiveness."[74]

Dr. Livingston was a giant in the world of pediatric epilepsy, writing four books and three hundred and fifty scientific articles in the field, as well as being a staunch advocate for

---

73 Samuel Livingston, "Childhood Epilepsy: An Overview, 1936-1973," *Pediatric Annals* 2, no. 8 (August 1973): 10-22.

74 Ibid.

the rights of people with epilepsy. In fact, he worked with Robert Kennedy to remove statutes discriminating against people with epilepsy in US immigration laws.[75]

MILLICENT KELLY

Livingston's close partner in this work was a registered dietician named Millicent Kelly. Kelly graduated from the Johns Hopkins School of Dietetics in 1949 and was hired at the nutrition clinic there. "Our job was to teach diets," she says. "Diabetic diets, low-calorie diets...whatever the patient needed. And that's where I learned about the ketogenic diet and met Dr. Livingston."[76]

When she first heard about dietary treatment for epilepsy, she "thought, my goodness, how could this be? But I learned how it could be." Others, however, weren't so enthusiastic. "Some of the dietitians would say, 'Oh, that awful diet,' because it was so restrictive, not realizing how effective it was."

"It wasn't a diet you could just read out of a book and have everybody follow it. It was individualized, and that's what the dietitian did." Her role was to help calculate macronutrients and tailor the diet to each individual child, accounting for the child's growth, nutritional needs, and more.

The intensity of this hands-on approach is one reason why the diet lost popularity over the time of Mrs. Kelly's career

---

75 "Samuel Livingston Dies," *The Washington Post*, August 25, 1984.

76 "Millicent Kelly and the Modern History of the Ketogenic Diet," The Charlie Foundation, April 24, 2018, YouTube Video, 8:47.

in favor of ever-expanding drug therapies. "It is far easier for parents and for the patients themselves to swallow one or several pills every day than to comply with such a rigorous diet. Compared with new, ever-developing medications, the diet came to seem like too much trouble."[77]

Other ketogenic centers across the country began to close, and the program at Hopkins shrunk, leaving Kelly and her colleagues "the lone slender threads that kept the ketogenic diet helping kids at Hopkins."[78] Dr. John Freeman would eventually say, "If Millie hadn't been around all these years, I think the diet would've been lost. Gone. That's how important she is."[79]

DR. JOHN FREEMAN

When Dr. Livingston retired from Hopkins in 1973 to enter into private practice, he handed the reins of pediatric epilepsy to Dr. John Freeman. Dr. Freeman had, during his residency, spent time at the seizure clinic at Columbia, "a clinic with too many patients seen only by residents and fellows, in too short a time, with minimal supervision," as he describes it in his 2007 memoir *Looking Back: A Career in Child Neurology*. "I resolved that our clinic at Hopkins would be different."[80]

77 John M. Freeman et al, *The Epilepsy Diet Treatment: An Introduction to the Ketogenic Diet*, (New York: Demos, 1994):33.

78 Jim Abrahams, "Mrs. Kelly," *Keto Lifestyle* (blog), The Charlie Foundation, accessed October 22, 2020.

79 "Millicent Kelly and the Modern History of the Ketogenic Diet," The Charlie Foundation, April 24, 2018, YouTube Video, 8:47.

80 John M. Freeman, *Looking Back: A Career in Child Neurology*, (Seattle: Book Surge Publishing, 2007): 219.

Dr. Freeman was known as not only a caring physician, but a staunch advocate for his patients. He was well-practiced in all forms of therapy for epilepsy, including pharmaceuticals. Still, when asked to speak at a conference on the physiology of epilepsy in 1992, he took the opportunity to remind the researchers "while the scientists are diddling in their labs, skewering cells in the hippocampus, or looking for these various channels of things, or whatever they do, kids are suffering, and their parents are, too...all we, as clinicians, can do is poison the kid's developing brain with these drugs, and the scientists haven't even been of any help to us in choosing the right drug."[81]

Dr. Freeman's concern over the harsh side-effects of drugs made him one of the few neurologists of his era to keep administering the diet long after others had stopped. He acknowledged "the diet *is* a lot of trouble. No one would dispute that. But if it works—if it works—as can loudly be heard from the parents for whom it is successful, it becomes not only tolerable, but '*amazing,*' '*fantastic,*' '*a miracle.*'"[82]

It was Dr. Freeman who, in 1994, was able to stop Charlie Abrahams's seizures. Perhaps the best way to convey Dr. Freeman's unique perspective, and the importance of the Jim and Nancy Abrahams to the importance of the ketogenic diet, is to share this story:

After Charlie's seizures stopped, his father put his Hollywood talents toward spreading the word. He shared his story with

81   Ibid., 231.

82   Freeman et al, *The Epilepsy Diet Treatment*, 33.

the producers of *Dateline NBC*, who did a primetime piece about the family. He created a film called *First, Do No Harm*, starring Meryl Streep, depicting a story of a family not unlike his own. He and Nancy started the Charlie Foundation to encourage research, to educate neurologists about the diet, and to publish a book with Dr. Freeman and Ms. Kelly about the diet.

The *Dateline* segment led to a surge of interest in the diet among parents—what Freeman in his memoir calls "The Deluge."

Still, the medical community seemed more hesitant to embrace the diet. In my interview with him, I asked Abrahams about his memories of the late Dr. Freeman. He told me, "I was always hugely frustrated because progress seemed so slow. Dr. Freeman would always counsel patience. So, one year on his birthday I sent him a copy of *McGelligott's Pool*, the Dr. Seuss book about having patience when fishing." In reply, Dr. Freeman sent back the following homage to the original, in print here for the first time (as far as I know):

McElligot's Pill

by Dr. John Freeman

P Is for patience, and patience is cool
Whenever you fish in McElligot's pool.

But P's also for patients, but there is a chill
When you try to swap diets for popping a pill.

For everyone knows, except for a few
That pills are the answer to what'er ails you.

Doctors love pills, and companies too,
To deliver the treatments and profits–It's true

But a diet made up of all buttery fat
To control someone's seizures–now who thought of that?

Popping of pills is the answer—what's more
If three doesn't work then you ought to take four.

And if four doesn't work, there's always one more
That's stronger and safer than something before.

Try bacon and cream,—no sugar—that's new,
They say ketosis will be better for you.

Now, everyone knows that fats are all bad,
Make cholesterol high. Look what they did to your dad.

We've taught all physicians and the public the view

That fats are pernicious, and ketosis too

These diets are probably just one of those fads,
And the hundreds of seizures—it's really too bad

But just 'round the corner there's another new pill,
And right behind that is another one–still.

So, stop preaching a diet that's mostly all fat,
Have patience, you patients, it can't really be true
That a high fat diet is better for you!

With apologies to Dr. Seuss.

DR. ERIC KOSSOFF

Today, Dr. Eric Kossoff is director of the Pediatric Ketogenic Diet Program and the Child Neurology Residency Program at Johns Hopkins, as well as a professor of neurology and pediatrics. He is widely recognized as the world's foremost expert on the ketogenic diet for childhood epilepsy. But this wasn't the case in 1999, when Kossoff was a fourth-year child neurology resident.

One day he ran into Dr. John Freeman, who at the time was in charge of the ketogenic diet program, in the hallway of the children's center at Hopkins. "He said, 'Hey Eric, come with me.' I said, 'I'm busy, I have to see another patient,' but he said, 'No, you should see my patient first.'"

Dr. Kossoff went to visit the patient, a young girl from another state, and her mother. "She had failed multiple medicines. She was wearing a helmet for seizures and had several drop seizures in the room." The girl was on three medications and had been fasting in preparation for starting the ketogenic diet in a day or so.

"Dr. Freeman asked me what I thought, and I said, 'I agree, she's a very tough case.' He said, 'Come back on Friday.'"

"Well, on Friday I met John and went back to see her. We walked back in the room, and she was a different kid. The helmet was gone, and she was a happy, bright-eyed girl without any seizures...Dr. Freeman had already weaned two of her three seizure medications.'"

The girl was likely suffering from Doose syndrome, a form of epilepsy that is particularly responsive to the diet.

"I was flabbergasted, shocked, and hooked after that point," Dr. Kossoff says. "At that moment, I decided to focus on the ketogenic diet for my research, my epilepsy fellowship, and later my neurology career."

DR. MACKENZIE CERVENKA
A few years later, Dr. Mackenzie Cervenka was brought into the field in a similar way. While completing her neurology residency at the University of Maryland, she decided to specialize in adult epilepsy and was accepted to Johns Hopkins as a fellow.

There, she met Dr. Kossoff. "I was so floored because I got accepted to Johns Hopkins for my fellowship, and then when I did get accepted, Eric approached me and asked if I wanted to do a study on the diet for adults." Laughing, she says, "I was like, 'Wait, is that even a thing?' At the time it was not at all a thing." Intrigued, she agreed right away. "I said, 'Well, of course I want to do that,' and I ended up publishing that paper with him."

In 2010 after she'd finished the fellowship, Dr. Cervenka was invited to join the faculty at Hopkins. Part of her goal was to open a full epilepsy diet center for adults, the first of its kind in the world.

"Initially, we opened our center with the thought we would see patients from Dr. Kossoff's pediatric center, we would transition them to adult care, and everything would be great. We opened the center, and the first two patients in the door were adults who had never been on diet therapy. They said, 'Well, why in the world can't I have this?' I said, 'There's no reason why you can't,' and so that's what we did."

In the ten years since, she has published numerous studies on the efficacy of the diet and treated hundreds of patients, with effectiveness rates rivaling the results seen elsewhere in children. She is now director of the Adult Epilepsy Diet Center and an associate professor of neurology. That center, just an hour from my home, is still one of the few places practicing the ketogenic diet for adults. And this, dear reader, is where your humble narrator re-enters the story.

CHAPTER 8

HELLO, BACON!

———

"I like your pin," Judy says. "Is that...bacon?"

Judy and I are sitting in the brightly lit office of Dr. Mackenzie Cervenka, director of the Adult Epilepsy Diet Center at Johns Hopkins. She is young and energetic, with a kind and welcoming demeanor that immediately puts me at ease. She is also wearing, on the lapel of her white lab coat, a shiny pin featuring two reddish-brown squiggles.

"Yep!" beams the doctor. "We love bacon around here." She goes on to talk excitedly about her latest supermarket find: a frozen pack of mini hot dogs wrapped in bacon. Just pop 'em in the oven and enjoy.

My eyes get wide. The heavens open up—angels sing. I have finally found the diet for me! All these years on the pick-a-diet Wheel of Fortune. All these years trying low calorie, low fat, points-counting, meal-timing, macros-tracking, hormone-optimizing, and every other crazy thing out there. All along, right in front of me, it was as simple as bacon weenies. (Or is it pigs-in-a-pig?)

I'm here for the orientation session for the center's clinic, an intervention in which adults with epilepsy follow a low-carbohydrate diet and monitor both their seizure activity and other vitals. I will officially become a patient of Dr. Cervenka, and for some reason, that excites me.

***

It's taken a while to get to this land of bacon-weenies. My seizure while driving left me shaken up. I'm a pretty low-key person, so it somehow feels too dramatic to call it a near-death experience. But if the shoe fits, I suppose...

My regular neurologist was underwhelmed. "I'm not too worried about it," he shrugged, handing me a prescription for an increased dose of the meds I was already taking. What a relief, I thought. The last thing I want to do is worry my neurologist.

So, for a few months I took the pill and waited. I tried not to think about it, as the always-useless advice went. When I had the seizure at work, six months later, and my neurologist's answer was to once again increase my dosage, Judy convinced me to call her brother-in-law Romer.

Romer, as it happens, is a neurologist himself, and one of the world's leading experts in neuro-critical care. When a stroke or heart attack cuts off blood supply to your brain, Romer is the guy you want to see. He graciously agreed to a phone call, where I told him all about what was going on. "What I want to know," he said, his scientific mind clicking away, "is what changed?"

***

What changed? Good question. He recommended I push for a new round of tests—an EEG and an MRI. He thought, but didn't say, something more serious could be going on (a tumor, for example...something fun like that).

When those tests came back healthy ("unremarkable," even), I breathed a sigh of relief. But I also continued to wonder: did anything in my life change to bring back my seizures? Something in my lifestyle? My diet? I'd been playing around with low-carb dieting as a way to lose weight, and I'd heard about Jim Abrahams and ketosis as a treatment for epilepsy, but I hadn't looked into it seriously. After all, I'd been seizure-free for a long time, so why rock the boat?

But this latest round of seizures—two in six months—and Romer's question was enough to push me further. So, as a reader, and as a person who's interested in health generally, I did what I always do: I geeked out. I started reading books, listening to podcasts, watching lectures, and eventually reading medical research that was way over my head. But I pushed on, inspired by one driving question: what, if anything, can I do to prevent seizures in the future?

So, by the time Romer mentioned Dr. Cervenka, I already knew her name. I called the clinic and managed to get an appointment for a few months away. Joanne, the center's administrative coordinator, told me they have been flooded with interest ever since keto and low-carb diets had gotten popular. "I feel bad for all those poor potatoes," she laughs, admitting she follows a low-carb diet herself. Every time I call, we chat and exchange recipe ideas. I feel like I'm talking with a friendly co-conspirator.

***

The orientation is a full day that includes appointments with Dr Cervenka and with Bobbie Henry-Barron, the clinic's dietitian. These Wonder Women are at the forefront of epilepsy research, and after months of *reading* their research, I can't wait to *be* their research.

Judy has taken the day off from work to join me here, which makes me happy. After all, I love to cook and she loves to eat what I cook. So, if I'm going to be cooking according to certain restrictions and rules, and I'm going to have to avoid certain temptations for the next year, it will be helpful for her to know what they are. More than this, though, she's here to keep me honest.

After meeting with Dr. C about my epilepsy, we sit down with Bobbie. She analyzes my food log for three days. Judy helpfully fills in the gaps, like those late-like snacks I somehow forget to mention. Bobbie is...impressed, shall we say, by the number of calories I'm eating. "Well, you are a big guy," she says, "and you do exercise..."

We then join the other participants in a small conference room for an education session. There's quite a variety of people here from all walks of life, and it strikes me how epilepsy takes so many forms and affects so many different people. Given how rare it is I meet another person with epilepsy, it's oddly comforting.

The session is informative and engaging, and by the end of it I can't wait to get started. Even Judy, whose upbringing in the Philippines taught her the motto "it's not a meal if it doesn't have rice," is willing to give this new way of eating a try.

GETTING MAD

So, what is this magic, bacon-weenie diet wielding the power to stop neurons at the speed of light? The clinic uses a variation of the ketogenic diet called the modified Atkins diet, or MAD.

Like regular Atkins (yes, THAT Atkins), it asks you to limit your carbohydrate intake to twenty net grams per day. ("Net" in this case means total carbohydrate minus fiber.) The "modification" is patients are not just *allowed* to eat fat, as Dr. Atkins advised, but actually *encouraged* to.

By the numbers, MAD looks like turning the standard, SAD diet on its head. About 64 percent of your calories come from fat, 30 percent come from protein, and only about 6 percent come from carbohydrates.[83] What does that look like on the plate? Here's a recommended dinner from Dr. Cervenka and her colleagues:

- Sliced chicken, coated in egg and low-carb baking mix then fried in olive oil.
- Steamed, mashed cauliflower with salt, pepper and butter (mashed "potatoes").

---

83 Kossoff et al, The Ketogenic and Modified Atkins Diets, 196.

- Half of a cup of strawberries topped with heavy whipping cream.[84]

MADness, right? Extreme? Dangerous? Fad-like? It all seemed pretty reasonable and doable to me. But why does it work?

YOUR BRAIN IS A HYBRID

It was surprising to me—as it is to most people—that a diet could affect the functioning of the brain. But why should it be? As psychiatrist Georgia Ede likes to say, "Studies have shown conclusively that the head is, in fact, part of the body."[85] Funny, isn't it, how we kind of forget that? We take it for granted our food affects our stomach, our heart, our muscles, and our bones, but we somehow believe the brain is a separate entity entirely. In fact the brain, though only weighing a few pounds, is an energy hog, consuming about 20 percent of our energy.[86]

It turns out my earlier analogy about Michael's car works for the brain, too. When there's glucose in the body, the brain will run on glucose. This is how most of us fuel our brains, stopping at the carbohydrate gas station every couple of hours to keep the hanger at bay.

---

84 Ibid., 191.

85 Georgia Ede, "Our Descent into Madness: Modern Diets and the Global Mental Health Crisis," Low Carb Down Under, April 21, 2018, YouTube video, 32:55.

86 Nikhil Swaminathan, "Why Does the Brain Need So Much Power?" *Scientific American*, April 29, 2008.

But it's also possible to run the brain on fat. Specifically, when fat is burned in the body, it produces a byproduct called ketones. These are the acids Dr. Geyelin and Dr. Wilder found in patients' urine. The brain can use these ketones as an alternative fuel source. As Dr. Cervenka explained in the clinic, "The brain loves ketones. It soaks them up."

Ketones are sometimes called a "less excitatory" source of fuel for the brain. In other words, the ketone-fueled brain is less likely to start misfiring. Here's another analogy: it's like burning a big, hardwood log in your fireplace instead of kindling. The kindling will light up fast and burn hot, but the log gives off low, steady, long-lasting heat.

Interestingly, doctors still don't know exactly why ketones have this effect on the brain. (Though this can also be said of many epilepsy medications.) It's an area of continuing research, and folks like Dr. Cervenka and Dr. Kossoff are getting closer to answers every day. This may be why the diet is still, in the neurology community, seen as a last resort, something on the far end of the treatment spectrum. Does it matter? Not to me. I resolved if this diet was a better way to fuel my brain and stood even a chance of protecting me against seizures, I was going to give it a try.

Since my new, amped up dosage of medication seemed to be keeping seizures at bay (knock on wood) and the side-effects weren't devastating, Dr. Cervenka suggested we use the diet as an adjunctive therapy—that is, in addition to, not instead of, the medication. This was just fine with me. The way I saw it, I was at war with this thing, and I was going to use every weapon in my arsenal to keep it in line. If this diet could contribute to keeping me seizure-free for years, then I was all in.

***

When I spoke with Jim Abrahams for this book, I mentioned it took fifteen years of living with epilepsy before I ever heard about the diet. His reply? "It's still grossly underutilized. The world's epilepsy population is around sixty million people. We know from published studies over half the people who try the diet have at least 50 percent seizure reduction. And for about 20 percent the seizures go away completely. So, you know, crunch those numbers and you get a lot of people who could benefit from the diet today."

Dr. Kossoff had a different perspective: "I can't deny there are certainly other places around the world—Africa, Southeast Asia—there are places where the diet could be used." But in the US, even if someone's regular neurologist doesn't use dietary treatment, "if the family wants it, they will find a way to get it."

Both of these are excellent points. Again, "Despite its proven efficacy...the ketogenic diet is still regarded as a 'treatment of last resort' by many neurologists and physicians who manage seizure patients."[87] In other words, after all else fails, try changing what you eat. That's the standard of care in epilepsy. After exhausting pharmaceutical and surgical options, when you're finally at the end of your rope, hey, give it a shot.

---

87   Kossoff et al, *The Ketogenic and Modified Atkins Diets*, 67.

What if we gave it a shot earlier? Maybe instead of and maybe in addition to those other therapies, depending on the case. This, I think, is what the late Dr. Freeman meant when he said in his memoir, "Decisions about treatment should be made by the family with the physician's advice, not by the paternalistic physician."[88]

Dr. Cervenka taught me a lot that day about my brain and my condition. Even though it's cliché to say knowledge is power, "empowered" is the best word to describe how I felt on the way home. The fear, the mistrust, the creeping sense of doubt—all the ways in which I'd been held hostage by my own brain—I won't say they evaporated, but the knowledge I gained in the clinic was the best ammunition yet. I couldn't wait to apply it to my own life.

---

88 Freeman, Looking Back, 228.

PART THREE

THE FAT-FUELED LIFE

CHAPTER 9

THE "MAGIC" DIET: THE POWER OF SERENDIPITY

———

Millicent Kelly remembers the children in her clinic saying, "I do well because I'm on my magic diet." For them and their parents, it must've seemed like a kind of sorcery to be able to eliminate their seizures and enable them to live life again. But the real magic, oddly enough, is often the luck that brings people to the diet in the first place.

Over and over, I had to ask myself: what are the chances? What were the chances I'd get epilepsy? Well, by the numbers, one in twenty-six. So, it's pretty rare overall, but even rarer I'd develop epilepsy at the age of twenty-eight since most diagnoses happen in children. What are the chances, when my car rolled off the road on a major highway, I'd walk away unscathed? And what are the chances I'd discover the ketogenic diet by listening to a weight-loss podcast, and I'd end up at a clinic working with one of the world's leading researchers? I can't imagine.

In my dozens of interviews for this book, one thing which came up again and again was the role of serendipity in the ketogenic journey.

***

Dr. Cervenka was kind enough to chat with me about her experience, and I asked her how she first became interested in this field. She said it was a chance encounter during her neurology residency. "I did my pediatric neurology rotation at Johns Hopkins. One day, I was in the hallway, and this random, lovely gentleman who worked in the ketogenic diet center came up to me and asked me if I liked the Counting Crows."

The man explained he had bought a ticket to a benefit featuring the singer of the Counting Crows that night, but he couldn't use it. That gentleman was Dr. James Rubenstein, a pediatric neurologist at Hopkins. "So, I went to this concert, and other than just wanting to go, I had absolutely no idea what the benefit was for. Before the concert started, this couple came up on stage told their story."

The couple was Gerry and Mike Harris. They found themselves in the emergency room at Hopkins when their five-month-old daughter Carson began suffering from infantile spasms, a very severe form of epilepsy. As the couple describe it, "Twelve hours, a spinal tap, and an EEG scan of her brain later we were told she has a rare form of epilepsy called 'infantile spasms.' There are no words to describe the emotions we experienced upon hearing the news our daughter had about a 20 percent chance of recovering." Gerry and Mike were offered a number of treatment options, including a regimen of steroids and heavy doses of medication. But they also saw Dr. Eric Kossoff, the foremost voice in dietary therapies for pediatric epilepsy today. Dr. Kossoff helped the couple to quickly get Carson on a ketogenic diet, and it worked. Carson's parents said, "We are overjoyed to report Carson is now developing normally and continues to be seizure free."

So moved was the couple that they started the Carson Harris Foundation, a non-profit with a mission "to increase awareness on the issues that affect individuals with epilepsy and raise funds in support of clinical and research efforts on the diagnosis of epilepsy and its treatment including, but not limited to, diets, surgery, and anticonvulsant medications." As it happened, this concert was a fundraiser for that foundation.

"What's interesting," said Dr. Cervenka, is that "I had never actually heard of it. As an adult neurologist, it was not taught to us in any way whatsoever. I didn't even know you could use diet as part of a treatment for epilepsy, and I was going into epilepsy as my chosen field in neurology. It's really hard to believe."

At the concert, she had a chance to meet Dr. Kossoff. "He seemed like this big celebrity to me," she laughed, "this doctor who had started this diet on this patient—I was like, 'oh my gosh!'" The rest is history.

***

Dr. Inna Hughes is another neurologist who came upon ketogenic diet therapy somewhat by chance. She got her medical degree at Washington University in St. Louis, then went on to complete a PhD in developmental biology.

Most medical students spend lots of time weighing their options and feeling out different fields of practice by trying them on for size during a number rotations over several years. But Dr. Hughes became hooked on neurology at the very start. "It was my first rotation, and there were some really amazing epileptologists at Wash U. They were just really cool people who were very excited."

At Washington, however, "They weren't all that interested in diet therapy," she says. "They had a small program, but it wasn't talked about much. Medical students didn't get much exposure to it." Rather, it was during her residency at the University of Rochester where she first encountered the ketogenic diet. When she discovered it, she again realized she had found her match. "I declared pretty much as early as I could that I was going to become an epilepsy specialist."

Epilepsy, she found, appealed to her innate love of fitting together bits of knowledge like a puzzle. "All the stuff I learned in undergrad science, every bit of weird trivia in biology and physics and math, and everything, and every bit of the medicine I learned in medical school, we use it every day in working with patients with epilepsy. It was very, very exciting to find a place where all that stuff that you stick up in your head for a later date actually had a use."

She encountered a child on diet therapy early on, "and it just kind of triggered an interest: 'Oh, we can use diet for care of epilepsy patients.'" Not that she was entirely surprised. "My parents were mildly disappointed I became a physician, I think, because they had lots of beliefs in alternative and holistic medicine. My dad fundamentally believes food is medicine. So those ideas of the use of food as medicine were not foreign to me. During my MD and PhD I rotated in places like GI labs. So again, the kind of information that came about ketogenic diet was just stuff that was partially in my head anyway, so it was kind of fun to put it together."

So, what are the takeaways from these stories? Both Dr. Hughes and Dr. Cervenka were young and starting out in their field which means they were naturally curious and had an openness to hearing new ideas and new perspectives. Sadly, not everyone has this inclination.

In a critique on *The New York Times's Well* blog, Dhruv Khullar, MD, describes the process of "pimping," a teaching technique commonly used in medical school. The senior doctor asks "a rapid series of questions, from thought-provoking and relevant to esoteric and unanswerable. It continues until teachers run out of questions, or doctors in training run out of answers. I'll let you guess which usually comes first."[89]

Pimping, says Dr. Khullar, is not just frightening but, "Medical training's emphasis on demonstrating how many facts we know—typically in front of colleagues, nurses, patients and

---

89 Dhruv Khullar, "Doctors Getting 'Pimped,'" *Well* (blog), *The New York Times*, May 26, 2016.

families—is problematic. It encourages us to learn to show, not grow." The concern can be lasting since, "Our training environment affects how we practice throughout our careers."

In other words, doctors are taught to memorize, not question, and to think factually, not critically. A rare physician can do both yet finding one can be a matter of luck.

***

Perhaps this is why for many patients, too, there is an element of serendipity in how they happen to find the diet. Jim Abrahams was looking in a medical school library for Lennox-Gastaut Syndrome, and it just so happened the "Ketogenic Diet" was alphabetically proximal. For Jon Landry, it was a lifelong friendship with Vinnie Tortorich.

When I interviewed Vinnie for this book, he mentioned off-handedly, "Jon is a childhood friend of mine, and he just started NSNG. He's also a guy with epilepsy."

I tracked Jon down that weekend and messaged him online, and he agreed to chat with me right away, "after I fix me another cup of coffee for the talk."

We each poured ourselves some coffee, and then we got on the phone. I could tell right away Jon is a kind, thoughtful man who speaks in the southern drawl of his native Louisiana. He told me he had a few seizures when he was very young, but he outgrew it for most of his childhood. Then, in his early twenties, he was in a car accident and the seizures came back, first as grand mals but then as petit mals, too.

He went on medication, which helped, but then he was offered the opportunity to be a test student at Louisiana State University's neurology clinic. He was one of the first to receive a Vagus Nerve Stimulator (VNS), a device installed in the patient's chest that can ward off seizures before they happen. Unfortunately, it didn't work.

He estimates for several years now he's had thirty to forty seizures a month. They were mostly petit mals, but every now and then he'd have a grand mal seizure as well. "They last only somewhere from one second to ten seconds, but they were ruining my day, I guess you could say. The problem was, stuff that was happening when I had seizures: falling down, hurting myself." He showed me a collection of gruesome post-seizure photos featuring black eyes, facial swellings, and even a huge gash in his head jaggedly stitched together. These photos are a reminder of how debilitating this disorder can be. "It was getting worse and worse, and it was upsetting my parents. They wanted me to get better. My friends wanted me to get better."

Jon's doctor at LSU offered to get him enrolled in a clinical trial for another new device. Similar to a pacemaker monitoring and responding to heart rhythms, the Responsive Neurostimulation for Seizures, or RNS, is a medical device able to monitor and respond to brain activity to prevent seizures from happening. "I said, 'Sign me up. I've got nothing to lose.'"

Right around the same time, he had a change of medication, and he also had an encounter with his childhood friend Vinnie Tortorich. "Me and Vinnie's brother Mike are like best friends, I guess you'd say. My mamma taught school with Vinnie's mamma, so it's a long family thing."

"One time, we went to eat out at a seafood restaurant, and Vinnie said, 'Jon, are you ready to lose that belly?' I was eating a seafood platter and I said, 'Vinnie, shut up. I could care less about losing my stomach. I like what I eat.'"

Jon's doctor had always talked to him about his weight, telling him it may be making his medication less effective. Then-nearlier this year, Mike finally decided to take his brother's advice about cutting out the carbs. "Me and Mike were picking Vinnie up at the airport and I said, you know what, Vinnie? I'm ready to start your diet. I'm ready to lose my stomach." So, Tortorich told him about NSNG.

All at once, Jon had a readjustment of the RNS device, a new medication, and he started the diet. When I spoke to him, it'd had been a few months since all these changes. Through this combination, he says, "I went from thirty or forty seizures a month, to five seizures the following month. And this month I had no seizures."

He called and told his neurologist about the success. She watched Vinnie's film *Fat: A Documentary* and agreed Jon should continue the diet. She suggested the success was due to all of these interventions complementing one another. "She said, 'It's everything. It's not just your medicine, it's not just putting this thing on your brain, it's a lot of stuff working together,' and she said that diet is helping my medicine flow through my body." With the combination of eating right, the RNS adjustment, and the new medication, "I'm getting eight to ten hours of sleep, I'm moving around more. I'm doing more stuff. I have a lot more energy. Three weeks—not even three weeks—after I started the diet, it just all got better."

I asked him what was hardest in making the switch from his favorite fried seafoods to NSNG. "Nothing, really. All you got to do is put your mind to it, and it didn't take anything to start doing it. And I can say, I'm very, very happy now—in a better mood every day and doing a lot more stuff." In the three months since starting, he's not only gone seizure-free, but he's lost forty-two pounds and gone from a size-forty-six waist to a size forty. "You could basically say it's like a miracle right now for me."

***

But the most powerful story of serendipity may be the one told by Jessyca Reynolds at the KetoCon 2020 virtual conference. Jessyca started a ketogenic diet in 2016, after years of battling depression, food addiction, and weight issues. "I was three hundred and nine pounds, I was miserable, and I was suicidal," she said, "and the ketogenic diet changed all that." She was able to improve not only her weight but also her mental health. Seeing this amazing transformation, her husband Mike joined her five months later and lost sixty pounds himself.

When their daughter Clara turned five years old, she started having seizures. "We almost lost her," Jessyca recalled, telling of Clara's second seizure. "Her little forty-five-pound body jerked and twisted. Bone and blood came from her mouth, and her bladder released. We were scared to death."

Clara continued to seize as she was being airlifted to the hospital and for several more hours, until she was given a paralytic and put on a breathing tube. Doctors didn't know whether there would be any lasting damage.

Her doctors put her on medication which, after several adjustments to the dosage, did stop the seizures. But it came at a high cost.

"Her personality changed," Jessyca said. "She became super withdrawn. She never wanted to go anywhere. She did not want to talk to friends at school. She cried every morning because she didn't want to go to school and be around people. It was just her new normal personality; she was afraid all the time."

This went on for nearly five years. Clara still had breakthrough seizures, such as when she was sick or had a fever, sometimes around friends or in public. "It was a really tough life for all of us." When Clara was nine, they were at a regular neurologist appointment. There they saw a framed flier on the wall for The Charlie Foundation mentioning diet and epilepsy. She went home and looked it up.

"I was shocked. We'd been using meds for five years, and in all that time no one had ever mentioned Clara's diet. We were pro-ketogenic, seeing all it had done for us," Jessyca said, "but we had no idea it could be used for epilepsy."

Clara knew her parents were keto, but she didn't want to do it herself. So, they began to slowly swap out higher-carb foods for lower-carb options, such as exchanging her bread for tortillas. Clara kept having breakthrough seizures, so they sat her down for a serious talk. They told her they were going to put her on the diet. "Clara cried," she said. "She cried a lot. It was not easy to break that news to her, but as a parent, I couldn't know there was something that might help her and not try it. That would have been irresponsible of me. It would have been wrong."

As parents, they made that decision, even though it was not popular with their friends, their parents, or anyone else in Clara's life. But they saw changes right away. "Clara blossomed. She had been in fourth grade and was reading at a fifth-grade level. After one year of eating keto, she tested at a 13.0 grade level—that's first year of college." She took up sports and cheerleading again. She began to go longer and longer without seizures and was weaned onto lower and lower levels of medication.

Now aged twelve, Clara has embraced the diet as her own. "I recently overheard her saying to one of her friends, 'even if my parents didn't make me do this, I'd still do it.'"

Jessyca only wishes they'd discovered the diet sooner. "Looking back, I think, 'Man, diet should have been the first line of defense, and then add meds if needed.'"

***

It shouldn't be this way. It's insane a long-established, proven treatment exists with the ability to help as many as 60 percent of people with epilepsy, but few actually learn about it. Doctors like Mackenzie Cervenka and Inna Hughes are changing that through their work. Jim Abrahams, Gerry and Mike Harris, and Jessyca Reynolds are changing it through their fundraising and speaking, and word is definitely spreading.

Of course, communication is a two-way street. How many times in life do we happen upon something but dismiss it before we give it a chance? How often does an idea seem too far-fetched, too far-removed from what we've been taught to be true? We need to be open to the ideas that come our way. It helps to be an outsider.

CHAPTER 10

MAVERICKS: THE POWER OF BEING AN OUTSIDER

"If four out of five people agree on something, listen to the fifth."

I heard this saying a few years ago, but I never understood it. Isn't this a democracy? Doesn't majority rule? If most people agree the sky is blue, why would I listen to the crazy guy who says otherwise?

Well, that depends. Is the crazy guy saying the sky is pink polka dots, or is he saying at some times of day, "Molecules and small particles in the atmosphere change the direction of light rays, causing them to scatter. Scattering affects the color of light coming from the sky, but the details are determined by the wavelength of the light and the size of the particle?"[90] In other words, he might not be crazy, but rather, he might

---

90 "What Determines Sky's Colors At Sunrise And Sunset?" University of Wisconsin—Madison, ScienceDaily. Accessed October 22, 2020.

know something the others don't. Also, if he's willing to fly in the face of what everyone else believes he must be pretty confident in that knowledge. For that reason, he's worth at least listening to.

I wouldn't call myself an outsider. I've been described as "easygoing," "affable," and even a "nice guy." Most of the time, I get along by going along. But opposites attract, and I've always enjoyed listening to the mavericks out there who see things their own way—the outsiders. When it comes to a field as wide-open as health, there's an advantage to being an outsider. Outsiders are open-minded. Outsiders are skeptical. Outsiders have nothing to lose.

***

Even though his book gives an insider's glimpse into the fitness industry, Vinnie Tortorich is a bit of an outsider. At college, his physical education degree required he take a number of pre-med classes, cheek and jowl with the aspiring doctors. "I was the kid in class who'd question everything," he said. "The other kids hated me because they just wanted to get A's and go on to med school. I'd raise my hand and they'd roll their eyes and say, 'here we go again.'"

One thing that struck him—particularly as a football player who was interested in exercise science—was human metabolism. "One week the professor would say, 'Fat is the body's preferred fuel source.' So, there's young Vinnie, dutifully scribbling down, 'Fat is the body's preferred fuel source.'"

"Then two weeks later, he says, 'If you want to do athletics, you need carbohydrates.' So I raised my hand, and said, 'Professor, I thought you just told us fat was the preferred fuel source.' He'd say 'Yeah, no, forget about that.'" His outsider status, along with his natural curiosity, gave him the opportunity to see things differently.

One day he was working in the lab, putting athletes through a brutal workout and measuring respiration, blood markers, and calorie expenditure. Afterward, he remembers his classmate offered him some M&Ms from a small, single-serving bag. "I turned the bag over and I said, 'Huh. This whole bag is only two hundred calories. We just had had that guy up in the gym, and he was about to throw up by the time we stopped that treadmill—he barely got over two hundred calories. So how in the hell can we tell people they can exercise the fat away?'"[91]

These early experiences set him apart from the trainers of the day through the carbo-loading and low-fat fads of the eighties and nineties. His skepticism made him an outsider within his own profession, and it's taken his profession thirty years to come around.

***

Speaking of "carbo-loading," Professor Tim Noakes, PhD, is another low-carb outsider in the world of nutrition—though he wasn't always that way. His bestselling book *The Lore of*

---

91 Brad Kearns, "Vinnie Tortorich—Fitness Confidential Author, Celebrity Trainer," October 30, 2018, *Get Over Yourself Podcast*, podcast, MP3 audio, 1:14:57.

Running was one of the key works to popularize the idea of pasta dinners for athletes in the nineties. But in 2010, at age sixty, Noakes had what he calls his "Damascene moment."[92]

The South African researcher had just finished a book about the dangers of over-hydration in distance running (another iconoclastic work that put him at odds with the majority of exercise scientists and drew the ire of Gatorade-maker PepsiCo), and he decided to go out for a run. Although a lifelong runner, he found himself struggling that day, thanks to his weight having crept up over the years. "Indeed, my forty-one years of running, including over seventy marathons and ultra-marathons, had taught me that, while running produces a wide array of physical and emotional benefits, weight loss is definitely not one of them."[93] It also failed to prevent him from being diagnosed with Type 2 diabetes.

As it happens, he received an email ad that day for a new book called *The New Atkins for a New You* by Dr. Eric Westman, Dr. Stephen Phinney, and Dr. Jeff Volek. He was "appalled that these supposedly serious scientists could allow their names to be associated with Dr. Robert Atkins. He was the madman who, in the 1970s, had encouraged us to eat more saturated fat and less carbohydrates, willfully misleading the world with his dangerous dietary non-science."[94] But Noakes also knew "all three doctors [Westman, Phinney, and Volek] are exceptionally good at what they do."

---

92 Tim Noakes and Markia Sboros, *Real Food On Trial: How the Diet Dictators Tried to Destroy a Top Scientist* (London: Columbus Publishing, 2019), Kindle.

93 Ibid.

94 Ibid.

He ran out to buy the book and started reading it immediately. He found the science to be sound, and "By lunchtime, I had read enough to make my Damascene decision: I would ignore my skepticism, ingrained by forty years of medical 'education,' and put the advice of Westman, Phinney, and Volek to the test."

The experiment was a success, and Dr. Noakes has since become one of the most authoritative voices in the low-carb community. He has even said in interviews, "If you've got *Lore of Running*, tear out the section on nutrition."[95]

He says, "I had two options: I could continue preaching these wrong and potentially harmful lies and maintain the scientific nutrition status quo, the so-called conventional 'wisdom,' or I could admit my errors, try to correct them, and deal with the consequences."[96] It is the rare academic who is willing to so publicly contradict his own work. But as he says, "I was just doing what any good scientist does when faced with incontrovertible evidence that contradicts a view, no matter how deeply held: I changed my mind."

Dr. Noakes is also a hero in the low-carb community for another reason. He has stood up to the purveyors of conventional wisdom and won. His book *Real Food on Trial*, written with journalist Marika Sboros, tells the story of how Dr. Noakes was censured by the medical board of South Africa, but in 2017, ultimately won the resultant week-long

---

95 Colin Seymour, "Tim Noakes: 'If You've Got Lore of Running, Tear Out the Section on Nutrition,'" *Gone for a Run* (blog), February 2, 2012.

96 Noakes, *Lore of Nutrition*.

hearing by conquering the vested interests of the nutrition world with science. The book shows how the Association for Dietetics in South Africa—an organization sponsored by companies like Coca-Cola and Kellogg's—threw everything they could at Noakes, but ultimately, he prevailed.[97]

***

One of the key witnesses in Dr. Noakes's hearing was author Nina Teicholz, who I think is perhaps the best example yet of the power of being an outsider.

Teicholz is a science journalist, speaker, researcher, and author of *The New York Times* bestseller *The Big Fat Surprise: Why Butter, Meat, and Cheese Belong in a Healthy Diet.* Her book has opened many eyes to the truth behind the role of saturated fat and cholesterol in the diet.

The book is a thick, exhaustively researched volume including over one hundred pages of footnotes and bibliography and, believe it or not, it's an absolute page-turner. In it, Teicholz uses a keen, critical eye to systematically dismantle a simple but ultimately erroneous idea: saturated fat is bad for you.

"Almost nothing that we commonly believe today about fats generally and saturated fat in particular appears, upon close examination, to be accurate," Teicholz says in the introduction.[98] And a close examination it is. Teicholz spent ten years

---

97   Sonia Mountford, "Why is Big Food in Bed with Dieticians? Follow the Money!" *BizNews,* May 30, 2015.

98   Nina Teicholz, *The Big Fat Surprise: Why Butter, Meat, and Cheese Belong in a Healthy Diet,* (New York: Simon and Schuster, 2014): 2.

researching this book, drawing on her wide-ranging background in biology, American studies, and investigative journalism, finding and analyzing the original studies on which the dietary guidelines are based, including reviewing the original data and speaking to many of the studies' authors, then reviewing documents and memos written by government officials and diving into what turned out to be a wild and lawless world called nutrition science.

"I'm a little obsessive-compulsive," Ms. Teicholz laughs as she speaks to me over Zoom from her home in New York. "I probably get that from my dad." Something she also got from her father was a love of science.

Her father was an engineer, she says, "and somebody who read deeply about science. We always talked about scientific ideas at home, and we had great respect for the process of science and intellectual thought and rigor." Both her parents, she says, are "incredibly straight, honest people," and she took it for granted scientists held themselves to those same high standards.

"I didn't realize until afterwards like how very straight and narrow they were, compared to what I saw in this world of nutrition. What I saw was just a world that seemed unhinged, from a scientific point of view. There was bullying going on. There was industry interfering in scientific research."

Her original assignment, when she started in the early 2000s, was an article for *Gourmet* magazine on this as-yet-unheard-of thing called "trans fats."[99] In the course of writing the article, she found there was a lot more to uncover. "Some of the researchers I spoke to had also been looking at other kinds of dietary fats, and they said, 'You know there's a much bigger story here about all fats. We really got it wrong on saturated fat, and we were very wrong to put vegetable oils in place instead of saturated fats. Vegetable oils are actually quite dangerous.'"

The deeper she dug, the more she found, to the point where she now says, "I think I can say unequivocally that this is true: that the world of nutrition and nutrition policy is far more influenced by politics, by ideological interest, and by money than it is by good science."

The Big Fat Surprise is a must-read for anyone who's interested in food and public health. I can't possibly do it justice here, but listed here are just a couple of truth-bombs to whet your appetite.

COCO-NUTS!

Ever wonder why coconut oil is good for you one minute and deadly poison the next? Ask your local soybean farmer. Ever since the 1930s, the American Soybean Association (ASA) has been locked in a war with coconut and palm growers from the Philippines and Malaysia. You may be thinking, "What's tofu got to do with it?" Think soybean *oil*, the

---

99   Nina Teicholz, "Heart Breaker," *Gourmet*, June 2004.

number-one edible oil in America. (Yum, yum!).[100] Until being banned in 2015, partially hydrogenated soybean oil was a key ingredient in everything from snack cakes, to crackers, to coffee creamer.

Strategies employed by the ASA to quash its Asian competition have included lobbying Congress for tariffs, printing racist ads and leaflets, and even funding research studies. The coconut and palm oil folks, meanwhile, fought back with lobbying, advertising, PR, and studies of their own.[101]

This still goes on today. A recent study in the *American Heart Association Journal* led to headlines all across the mainstream media warning of the dangers of coconut oil. Who paid for it? The California Walnut Commission; Ag Canada and Canola Oil Council; and The National Cattlemen's Beef Association.[102] In other words, lots of people who would be happy to see folks eat something other than coconut oil.

If you've ever been confused by the dizzying back-and-forth of headlines alternately vaunting and vilifying things like coffee, red wine, chocolate, and more, all you need to do is adopt actor Hal Holbrook as your own Jiminy Cricket and let him chirp in your ear: "follow the money."

Crazy conspiracy-theory? A 2007 review found nutrition studies funded by a food company were four to eight times

---

100 M. Shahbandeh, "US Consumption of Edible Oils by Type 2019," Statista, January 30, 2020.

101 Teicholz, *The Big, Fat Surprise*, 236.

102 Robyn O'Brien, "Widespread Panic and Coconuts: Follow the Money," *Robyn O'Brien* (blog), June 21, 2017.

more likely to find results favorable to the sponsor than ones not.[103] A good rule of thumb is if you read an article about a "new study" focusing on a single food or ingredient, skip it and head for the funny papers. Or at the very least, take it with a big grain of Mineral-Rich Mediterranean Sea Salt.

SWARTHY MEDITERRANEANS

Speaking of which, what about the Mediterranean Diet have I heard so much about? Surely the research on it is untainted. Teicholz has done some heavy lifting here, too. In a fifty-page, one-hundred-and-fifty-footnote chapter, *The Big Fat Surprise* gives an eye-opening history of the Mediterranean Diet (or Mediterranean Eating Pattern as it's now called by US Dietary Guidelines today). Some fun highlights?

The "capital 'D' Diet" was created in the eighties when two doctors, Antonia Trichopoulou from Greece and Anna Ferro-Luzzi from Italy, nostalgic for their disappearing culinary traditions sought to quantify just what was the healthiest diet for the people of their countries.[104]

The Diet was codified by vegetarian-leaning Harvard professor Walter Willett in 1993 with the creation of the Mediterranean Diet Pyramid. It included lots of grains, fruits, veggies, beans, legumes, and nuts, and way up top, where you almost can't see it, a tiny bit of lean red meat.[105]

---

103 Alison Moodie, "Before You Read Another Health Study, Check Who's Funding the Research," *An Apple a Day* (blog), *The Guardian*, US Edition, December 12, 2016.

104 Teicholz, *The Big, Fat Surprise*, 175

105 Ibid., 187.

The Diet was promoted relentlessly through a blitz of conferences in the nineties funded by—wait for it—the International Olive Oil Council. Teicholz details how doctors, researchers, and nutrition writers (so-called "Olive-Oil Ambassadors") enjoyed lavish, all-expenses-paid trips to beautiful Mediterranean climes.

She quotes the romantic descriptions used to sell the diet back home, including images of "handsome, rugged, kindly and virile" Greek laborers "enveloped in a rich lavender aura from the Aegean sea and sky." Heady stuff for the *American Journal of Cardiology*![106]

For a Mythology Diet (see Chapter 2) that's been through a dizzying number of versions and iterations, it's done pretty well for itself. It's been the subject of six hundred and fifty articles in *The New York Times* (and counting).[107] It's now one of three eating patterns endorsed by the US Dietary guidelines, and you'd be hard-pressed to find a family doctor who'd say a word against it. But doctors tend to like "evidence-based medicine." If it hasn't been proven in a clinical trial, it's not worth much.

CAUSATION VERSUS CORRELATION

Here's the thing: clinical trials are expensive, and, when it comes to food, nearly impossible to control. You can control whether a person takes a pill or a placebo for several months. You can't control what they eat all day, every day within the

106 Ibid., 191.
107 Ibid., 197.

same period. Nevertheless, Teisholz showed how "in the absence of trial data, as we'll see again and again over the last fifty years of nutrition history, epidemiological evidence has therefore been made to suffice."[108]

What's epidemiological evidence? It's a fancy term for observational studies, which in turn is a fancy term for: look at a bunch of people over time, see who becomes sick and who doesn't, and figure out what the sick people did differently than the healthy people. It's a very useful kind of study if you want to figure out, say, how COVID-19 is transmitted, but not very useful for slow-developing, multi-factorial diseases like diabetes, obesity, and heart disease. These studies often rely on food frequency questionnaires ("How many times do you drink skim milk in the average week?") which can be only as reliable as people are meticulous, trustworthy, and serious (and, come on, have you *met* people?). Also, it's hard to separate out the other factors—exercise, stress, relationships—with the potential to influence the outcome. As Teicholz says, these studies can "show only an association, not causation."[109]

Not that there have never been clinical trials for the Diet. Teicholz dissects two major trials from 1994 and 2006 often cited in support of the Diet. She proves these studies only "show how far nutrition experts will stretch the evidence to bolster support for a favored hypothesis."[110]

---

108 Ibid., 44.

109 Ibid., 42.

110 Ibid., 209.

The largest, most well-designed trial, though, was a 2008 Israeli intervention study, which showed quite definitively the Mediterranean Diet outperformed the low-fat diet on both weight loss and heart health. However—and this is the really wild part—the low-carbohydrate, high-fat diet outperformed them both.

SCIENCE CRUSADER

In the time since the book's publication, Teicholz has done anything but let up. She now heads the nonprofit Nutrition Coalition, whose mission is "to ensure the federal government's nutrition advice is based on comprehensive, systematic reviews of the most rigorous nutrition science available and to encourage additional research where that science is lacking."[111]

She has spent the last several years tirelessly leading letter-writing campaigns, meeting with congresspeople, writing articles, and giving interviews in an attempt to wrest control of the US Dietary guidelines from special-interest groups. It's been an uphill battle. The 2020 committee has many members with conflicts-of-interest, including ties to the food and pharmaceutical industry, or histories of promoting philosophies like plant-based diets.[112]

***

---

111 "Who We Are," Nutrition Coalition, accessed October 22. 2020.

112 "Who's on the Guidelines Committee" Nutrition Coalition, updated March 6, 2019.

And what *about* that plant-based diet? I've heard a lot about it lately. They say it's better for you and better for the planet. It turns out that exact phrase comes from EAT Lancet, a massive 2019 study involving a group of scientists from around the globe and led by Walter Willett of Mediterranean Diet fame. The report, which purports to be "the first full scientific review of what constitutes a healthy diet from a sustainable food system, and which actions can support and speed up food system transformation," suggests cutting back on meat, eggs, and dairy, and eating more fruits, vegetables, grains, legumes, and nuts—lots and lots of nuts.[113]

The report was promoted with a celebrity-studded launch event across forty cities, including PR pushes to newspapers and magazines around the globe—unusual fanfare for a scientific study. Who paid for all this? FReSH (Food Reform for Sustainability and Health), an organization whose list of backers includes a veritable who's who of "plant-based" junk food (PepsiCo, Nestle, Kellogg), pharmaceuticals (Bayer, Dupont), agricultural products (BASF, Cargill), and food additives (Unilever, Givaudan). So maybe, just maybe, some of these big companies have an interest in our eating (and, more to the point, buying) more plants.

Teicholz, a former vegetarian herself, finds it disheartening vegetarians and vegans, "who are pure of heart and sometimes ideological, are being used by a set of corporate interests."[114]

---

113 "The EAT-Lancet Commission on Food, Planet, Health," EAT Forum, accessed October 23, 2020.

114 Bret Scher, "Diet Doctor Podcast #21—Nina Teicholz," June 4, 2019, in *Diet Doctor Podcast*, podcast, MP3 audio, 56:05.

It's worth noting the World Health Organization (WHO) dropped its sponsorship of EAT Lancet after questions arose about the validity of the scientific basis for the diet.[115] Oh, and Walter Willett, the study's lead author, retired Harvard professor, Mediterranean Diet guru and probably the most powerful guy in the nutrition field today? The Nutrition Coalition has published a seven-page report detailing his various potential conflicts-of-interest, including hundreds of thousands of dollars he and his labs have received over the years from the nut industry.[116] That's a lot of nuts.

HEALTHY SKEPTICS

It's clear to me, even through a video call, Nina Teicholz is more than merely "a little obsessive-compulsive." What drives her is a belief in the principles of science, inquiry, and intellectual integrity. I asked her—for those of us who don't have degrees from places like Stanford and Oxford, who don't have a background in science or the discipline of an investigative journalist—what it takes to follow her example, to develop the kind of healthy skepticism needed in order to, well, stay healthy. Has she found, in her experience with the low-carb community, it's a certain type of person who is attracted to this idea: keto, low-carb, managing health through diet?

"That's a very interesting topic," she says. "Who's open to it, who isn't? It's becoming a lot more common as time has

---

115   Ingrid Torjensen, "WHO Pulls Support from Initiative Promoting Global Move to Plant Based Foods," *BMJ* 365, (April 9, 2019): 1700.

116   Bret Scher, "Diet Doctor Podcast #21."

gone on, and people see that it works. But initially the people who could entertain these ideas were more kind of outsiders, maverick kind of personalities. Someone who's outside the system a little bit, who's not invested in any institution,"

This is perhaps why she and Gary Taubes, science journalists, not traditional scientists, have become some of the preeminent voices in the low-carb community. "It doesn't matter if we piss people off, and our minds are more open to things."

***

Teicholz's work was a huge relief to me, being a large man of a certain age. I'd always been taught saturated fat and cholesterol were deadly killers. I worried that my brain-healthy diet might be heart-unhealthy, that I might be robbing Peter to pay Paul.

But that never sat right with me, either. After all, why would Mother Nature design a creature whose two major organs thrived on vastly different diets? As the so-called thinking animal, humans are the only animals who think about what they eat. Other creatures just, well...eat. And the things they eat give them the best possible chance of survival. (Have you ever seen a fat deer or a hypertensive lion?)

The Big Fat Surprise set my mind at ease about this conundrum, and I counted myself happy to be an outsider when it came to conventional wisdom.

There's a larger lesson here, I think. To question the status quo takes a kind of skepticism. To listen to a new way of thinking takes a lot of open-mindedness. But that's a difficult needle to thread: too skeptical and you begin to distrust everyone on everything, yet too open-minded and you're liable to fall for anything.

How do you strike a balance? Maybe the answer is to think like a science journalist. Follow a hunch but trust the evidence. Teicholz says, "I think for most people, part of what brings them along to a lower-carb diet is biological: they feel a lot better. They lose their taste for sweets. Their palate shifts over, and there's this positive reinforcement cycle of just feeling so much better. So many people say, 'I just cannot go back to feeling the way I used to feel.' Or maybe they get off their medications. There are such dramatic stories of transformation, and you hear them again and again."

More than anything, this book taught me to think critically about nutrition advice and to open my eyes to all that which can't be unseen. It's been tremendously freeing, to be able to observe the "next big thing," be it turmeric, açaí, flaxseed, or goat-milk kefir—or even ketone supplements—through this lens of healthy skepticism. I'm no longer chasing health up and down the grocery aisles, drinking fruit smoothies one minute and bulletproof coffee the next.

***

To put it even more simply, I like to ask myself a rhetorical question Dr. Fung posed on a podcast: *"What problem are you trying to solve?"*

He had just dispensed the advice that people trying to lose weight should avoid orange juice because of its high sugar content. The interviewer interrupted: "But what about vitamin C?"

"Are you suffering from scurvy?" Dr. Fung fired back. "If you're malnourished, then yes, drink the orange juice. But if you're trying to lose weight, juice is not your friend." The question we often lose sight of, he explained, is this one: "What problem are you trying to solve?"

I love this question. Ernest Hemingway once said a writer must have "a built-in, shockproof, shit detector."[117] These days, I think the same is true for a reader—particularly when it comes to health advice. Dr. Fung's question, for me, is a reliable shit detector. It helps me to navigate the muddy, manure-rich field of nutrition advice and find the stuff that's actually useful.

We should all be eating açaí berries from the Brazilian rainforest because they are packed with antioxidants. Why? Am I suffering from a lack of antioxidants? Red wine has resveratrol. Okay, but am I resveratrol-deficient? The question, "What problem are you trying to solve?" helps to toss out the crap and focus on the stuff that matters.

Tortorich, Noakes, Teicholz, Fung...all of their stories illustrate the power of being an outsider. They're open-minded, they're skeptical, and they act like they've got nothing to lose.

---

117 Stephen Miko, "The River, the Iceberg, and the Shit-detector," Criticism 33, no. 4 (1991): 503-25.

Perhaps by thinking like a science journalist—follow your hunch but trust your evidence—we can be outsiders, too.

CHAPTER 11

STUBBORNNESS: THE POWER OF PERSISTENCE

———

Gillian Szollos is speaking to me from her home in Canada, where she lives with her family, pets, and, well, chickens. I tell her I've always wanted to try the whole urban farming thing in our tiny backyard. "It's so worth it," she says, "it really is. Especially in this time of COVID, just to be able to have the therapy of going out and hanging out with your chickens. They're so curious and smart; actually, they're pretty intelligent creatures, and the eggs, oh my gosh—the best eggs ever."

"And of course," she adds, "we go through a lot of eggs in this house." Which brings us to why I have called. I have to start out by thanking Gillian for sharing her story so generously in podcasts and conference talks. It's a heartbreaking example of the importance of lifestyle in health.

Diagnosed with epilepsy as a child, Gillian had—like many children—outgrown it by her twenties...or so she thought. One day, at age forty-four, she was driving home from a busy day and experienced an aura, often the start of a full-blown seizure. It had been decades, though, since her last seizure, and so (in what she confesses, in hindsight, was a moment of bad decision-making) she decided to ignore it.

Two days later, having just been picked up by her husband for a lunch date, she was overcome by a much stronger aura. She remembers her mouth filling with saliva, an inability to speak, her hand jerking to the left, and her head dropping. After thirty years, the stalker of epilepsy had returned to her life. After a CT scan, MRI, and EEG, she was sent home with a renewed diagnosis of epilepsy and a prescription for Keppra.

"My life started to crumble," she says. She began to have five to ten seizures a day. The return of her seizures meant she could no longer drive, which was a hardship, living in the country with little access to public transportation. At work, she had just put together a massive program and was fully responsible for it. Even working from home, the constant seizures made it hard to keep up the pace at work. "I could no longer manage my responsibilities for my husband and my company."

Not only did the medication fail to stop her seizures, it came with enormous side effects on her mental and emotional health. "I was crying every day," she says. "That 'Keppra rage' you hear about? That's real, and it frightened me. It frightened my husband, and it frightened my daughter. The more the sadness and the rage overtook me, the more trapped I felt."

Gillian's family did their best to support her; her mother-in-law stayed with her during the day to monitor her seizure activity, and her husband took over more of the responsibilities both in their company and in the household. "He wasn't sleeping," she says, "How could he? Every time I moved in my sleep, he thought I was having a seizure—and often I was—so he'd wake up, stroke my head, and talk me through it."

The next morning, he'd wake up and go to work, exhausted. "I felt so guilty," she says, "epilepsy was taking so much from us."

She began to track everything—her medication, her seizures (by day and by time of day) her monthly cycles, and more. She noticed her seizure frequency tracked with her monthly period. She also noticed every time her Keppra dosage was raised, she'd have a few days seizure free, but then the next seizures would be terrible.

Then one night, it all came to a head. After a minor argument, Gillian snapped. As she put it, "The rage swelled like a tsunami." She ran outside in the cold with no coat or hat, and it took forty minutes for her husband to find her. "And when he did," she says, "I was on a bridge, looking down at the icy water, willing myself to jump."

Her husband took her home, wrapped her in warm blankets, and put her to bed. That night, he did something unusual: he opened a Facebook account. "It's important you understand what an introvert my husband is, to fully appreciate that gesture," she says. "He went online and joined every seizure support group he could find."

In one of those groups, he found the ketogenic diet. He told her about it the next morning, and she decided she would look into it. "I like research," she says, "and I decided I was going to figure it out." Since she was already a healthcare worker, she knew her way around a medical paper. She read everything she could find on the ketogenic diet and epilepsy and went to her neurologist with this new idea.

"He laughed at me and said that it only works on kids," Gillian tells me, incredulous to this day. Undeterred, she spoke to her family physician, who had never heard of keto, but who was at least willing to order the lab tests she needed to do it safely. "I started looking in my community to see if I could find a dietician who might be able to help me sort out my macros, get the maximum amount of micronutrients...nobody."

"But help was on its way," she says, "in the form of the internet." She found Dr. Eric Kossoff, who was willing to speak with her for an hour on the phone and point her to the resources from The Charlie Foundation and others.

She started on a strict ketogenic diet—90 percent of calories from fat—and in two weeks, her seizures stopped. "So, armed with all of my graphs and all of my charts, I went to my doctor and I said this Keppra is stopping today. It is killing me." The doctor suggested a switch to Tegretol, a medication Gillian had been prescribed as a young woman, which had left her with severe cognitive and memory impairments.

She did as she was told and filled the prescription, but she never started it. She stayed on the diet and went forty-nine days without a seizure. On that forty-ninth day, which was right before her period, she had an aura. "I decided to treat my implementation of the ketogenic diet like a science experiment." So, she did some more research, cut everything estrogenic out of her diet, and carefully monitored every single carbohydrate during specific points in her cycle. This did the trick.

"I didn't have another seizure," she says. "It really works."

Gillian is now six years seizure- and medication-free. Her story is a great example of the particular kind of focus it takes to find and embrace lifestyle treatment for disease. In many ways, she was ahead of her doctors in this area. When I spoke with her, though, she was careful to reinforce the importance of working with your doctor. "I really believe very passionately that from a therapeutic angle, you really need a primary care provider involved. It's important to be able to look at the bloodwork and to say, 'Okay you know what? Not only is my epilepsy better controlled than it was before, but all of these other markers of health are also improving.' That's a wonderful thing to be able to collaboratively document."

One reason this is so important is every person is different. "Your epilepsy is not the same as my epilepsy," she says, "and your ketogenic diet is probably not the same as my ketogenic diet. I think that when, especially people with epilepsy are going to give this a try, it is very important to go full on at first—minimum three-to-one, but preferably a four-to-one ratio [of fats to other macronutrients] to start. If you're achieving success, you can back off from there."

Gillian's perspective of treating diet as an experiment on yourself also includes a focus on tracking. "It's so important to track and to log—not just seizure activity, but also your blood sugar, how you're feeling, any changes in medication." This is its own form of persistence, and it could take a certain kind of person to succeed at it. "I'm very interested in research, and in evidence-based practice. These are sort of some fundamental core beliefs that I have. That really allowed me, I think, to have the success that I have."

***

Jennifer, who goes by her Twitter name "Seizure Salad," didn't have the opportunity to partner with her doctor in the same way. She began having temporal lobe seizures at age twelve. When she has a seizure, she says, "everything I'm looking at is like a dream, but it's happening in real life. My brain is telling me that I'm going to be able to predict, that everything that happens around me has happened before. It's very bizarre. I break out into a sweat and all my muscles get really warm. I'll get hand tremors, my fight-or-flight system kicks in for no reason."[118]

The doctors started her on Tegretol and told her to come back in three months for blood work to, perhaps, up the dose. "And this was kind of the model for my treatment for the next twenty years," she says. "I would go in, still having seizures. 'Okay, let's up your dose.' We'd up the dose—still

---

118 Brian Lenzkes and Tro Kalayjian, "Episode 26: Seizure Salad," April 3, 2019, in *Low Carb MD Podcast*, podcast, MP3 audio, 50:20.

having seizures. 'Okay, let's try this other medication.' And on it went."

She had read about the ketogenic diet and even mentioned it to her neurologist, who discouraged her, out of concerns about cholesterol, and told her they'd treat it as a last resort. After more medications, more EEGs, and more tests, a neurologist suggested a temporal lobectomy: the removal of a golf-ball-sized chunk from her brain.

She declined. "Given my history with this, and the last twenty years of these failed medications and the endless MRIs and EEGs, I was getting to be very 'done.' I got to this point where I just didn't care anymore. If I have seizures for the rest of my life, that's fine. I'm just tired of being a guinea pig."

She again mentioned the ketogenic diet and asked if it was something they could try, but the doctor emphasized the low adherence rate. They instead put her on a combination of Lamictal and Topamax, which affected her work and came with strong side effects. "It basically turned me into an idiot."

Another of those side-effects was panic attacks, for which she then had to take Paxil and Xanax, not to mention Ambien to help her sleep. "It was like this pharmaceutical avalanche," she says. One day when she was on the bus on the way to work she says, "part of my face stopped working." Panicked, she called a friend, who met her and took her to the hospital, where she learned the paralysis was merely a side effect of all the medication she was taking.

By the time she was forty-one years old, her doctor put her on Keppra, which didn't give her bad side-effects, but nor did it control her seizures. Her doctor wanted to raise the dosage to 3500 mg—a dose that's actually higher than the published guidelines. Not only that, but she had read Keppra can cause acute kidney disease, even at moderate dosage levels. "I was just like, 'Okay, this has got to stop. I can't do this anymore.'"

Like Gillian, she threw herself into research online and found The Charlie Foundation. She gathered all the information she could, bought a food scale, and went to a diet of 80 percent calories from fat, 15 percent from protein, and 5 percent from carbohydrates. "It was challenging, at first, to get that much fat in my diet," Jennifer says, "but I was determined. My doctor said there's a low adherence rate, and I just took that as a challenge. I was like, 'You know what? I'm gonna do this.' I don't want someone telling me what I can't do."

Within one month she was seizure free, and she still is today, two years later. "It blew my mind something so simple as diet was able to rein in symptoms that had been through tests, and medications, and all of this for so long. And despite all the doctors' best efforts through science and pharmaceuticals, that diet was able to take care of all of it."

Now she uses Twitter to spread the word about keto. "It frustrates me doctors automatically assume everyone's going to go with the path of least resistance. That it's just easier for me to be on a medication than to change my diet. You can't make a blanket statement that everyone's going to respond that way. Give them the opportunity. If they try it and it doesn't stick, that's on them. The physician should give them all possible treatment options and let the patient decide whether they want to eliminate carbohydrates or have brain surgery."

Jennifer herself admits that it was unwise to go it alone, and doesn't advise that you follow her example (nor do I). Her story illustrates the kind of desperate measures people are willing to take to get this important therapy. Thankfully, there's a growing awareness of the ketogenic diet, and it's becoming easier to find a practitioner through resources like The Charlie Foundation (*www.charliefoundation.org*).

***

The low adherence rate Jennifer's doctors worried about is a real issue for many patients, and there's a reason for it. Keto is hard—for both the patient and the doctor. When food is medicine, a person has to practice a great deal of care with what one eats and be thoughtful about every bite they put in their mouth.

Dr. Kossoff points to this difficulty as one of the reasons why, despite the growing mainstreaming of the diet, it's not more popular than it is. "In pediatrics, at least, there are no centers that don't believe in it. Everybody wants a ketogenic diet center. But there are neurologists who feel, 'I don't have the time, I don't have the energy, maybe I'm not good at it...' It's unfortunate." But the fact is, for a practitioner, it's hard work. It takes collaboration across disciplines, monitoring of a number of health markers, flexibility, and patient buy-in. "It's just hard," he says.

Hard, but to patients like Gillian and Jennifer, it's worth it. "Changing my diet was a lot cheaper than brain surgery," Jennifer laughs, "or even the thousand dollars a month that it costs for some medications."

Gillian says, "I am medication-free, I am working again, and I am happy again."

CHAPTER 12

TEMPERING THE TANTRUM: THE POWER OF MINDSET

———

"People don't get fat from overeating food." This bold statement from Robert Cywes, MD, PhD, snaps me out of the lull of my morning commute. "People get fat because they are addicted to a drug called carbohydrates."

In the course of three episodes of her *Diet & Health Today* podcast, author and researcher Zoë Harcombe, PhD, interviews Cywes on his great success in getting patients thin and healthy.[119]

Cywes is a bariatric surgeon, so for his patients, losing weight is the easy part. Bariatric surgery has a very high success rate in the short term. The problem is, the long-term results

———

119 Zoë Harcombe, "Carbohydrate Addiction—Part 1 With Dr. Robert Cywes," *Diet & Health Today,* June 6, 2018, podcast, MP3 audio, 34 min.

are not so hot.[120] Many people regain the weight after a few years, as they slip right back into old habits. Cywes's solution is to follow up the surgery with ongoing support in what he calls "AA for fat people." (As a former obese person himself, he feels comfortable using the very un-PC term "fat person," he says.)

Cywes explains food gives us two things: nutrition (fuel for the body) and endorphins (feel-good chemicals in the brain). Carbohydrate-rich foods like ice cream and potato chips are not very good at the former, but they're excellent at the latter.

This is why, when we feel a good ol' fashioned snack attack coming on, we're most likely to reach for something carb-filled. Cywes believes "a snack is always an emotional event," prompted not by the body's nutritional needs, but the brain's need for a break from stress or a change in mood. He makes the following parallel: in the old days, you'd get off a tough phone call at work and give yourself a break by stepping out for a smoke. Nowadays, you stop at the candy jar on the receptionist's desk instead. Unfortunately, although carbs are great at giving us the endorphins we crave, they're also uniquely good at causing us problems, like weight gain, diabetes, heart disease, Alzheimer's, and so on.

Cywes's clinic, then, is focused on teaching people to deal with their stress and emotions with endorphin-releasing *activities*, like playing music, meditating, or exercising, rather

---

120 "Long-Term Followup of Type of Bariatric Surgery Finds Regain of Weight, Decrease in Diabetes Remission," *The JAMA Network Journals ScienceDaily,* August 5, 2015.

than with endorphin-releasing *substances*, like a pint of Ben & Jerry's or a glass of wine.

The key word, he says, is capital-E Effort. Unlike substances, activities require effort we can get lost in for a while, giving the mind some space to process our stress. The feeling of accomplishment we get from our good work provides feel-good chemicals in the brain called endorphins. Substances, by contrast, will give a quick shortcut to the endorphins, but they will only mask those bad feelings, which pop up again later on.

The interview made me reconsider many of my habits, from the parade of hot K-cups that get me through my mornings to the after-dinner nibbles in front of the TV. Are all those habits merely little emotional crutches to get me through my day? That mid-afternoon handful of peanuts—am I really hungry, or just looking to delay a difficult work decision? Would a walk around the block be a better way of processing the situation? I began to wonder.

***

The psychological minefield around eating is something Jillian Holt knows well. In her mid-thirties, she started experiencing the aches and pains most people associate with aging. She'd see her doctor, walk away with a diagnosis of tendonitis or bursitis, and "get a cortisone shot here or there," but she began to grow frustrated that there were no real answers about the underlying cause of her pain with no indication of a better future.

She sought out a functional medicine doctor, who ran a comprehensive blood panel, and was shocked. She got a diagnosis, all right: with blood sugar levels above 400 (normal is considered less than 100) and an A1C, glycated hemoglobin, of 12 percent (below 5.7 percent is normal), it was Type 2 Diabetes. Her doctor put her on Metformin right away. "They actually re-ran the blood work. They said, 'This can't be right. You should be in a diabetic coma; you shouldn't be here having a conversation with me.'"

As it happened, she met up with an old friend the very next week. "I hadn't seen him in a while, and I saw that he had lost a lot of weight. I was like, 'What are you doing? You look terrific!'"

He told her about the ketogenic diet and how it had helped him to not only lose weight, but to help get his blood sugar under control. She looked into it and started eating strict keto right away.

Type 2 Diabetes is, in essence, a disease of dysregulation of blood sugar in the body. The body can't produce enough insulin to handle and store the sugar in the blood. Drugs like Metformin work by reducing the amount of sugar the liver releases into the blood, allowing the body's insulin system to handle the load imposed on it.

Jillian took the Metformin her doctor prescribed, but with a strict ketogenic diet, she also reduced the strain on her system by taking in a lot less sugar in the first place. It worked. "Within six months, my A1C went from 12 to 7.8, and my blood glucose was consistently in the 100–130 range."

The experience got her to start to think differently about food. "It really opened the door for me to start thinking about my health and the changes I could make with diet. I started thinking, what else can I do?" Despite getting her diabetes in control, she still experienced the joint pain that drove her to seek help in the first place. She ended up with a diagnosis of psoriatic arthritis, an extremely painful condition in which the immune system creates inflammation that can lead to swelling, pain, fatigue, and stiffness in the joints.

She began what's called an elimination diet protocol. After three months of cutting out foods like dairy, nightshade vegetables, and nuts, she was able to lower her SED rate (a blood marker of inflammation) from a 56 to an 8—well within the normal range of 0–22.

But one of the most important things she learned—and continues to learn—to heal is her emotional relationship with food. "When my youngest was about five, some stuff from my childhood resurfaced, and that's when my carbohydrate addiction kicked in. I would start sneaking a candy bar here or there, stopping by a drive-thru...and that's when I gained fifty pounds in about two years."

She now uses a more carnivore-style diet (and yes, that's just what you think it is) to help heal—not just her blood sugar and inflammation, but her emotional eating as well. "As Robert Cywes says, it's not really 'food addiction,' even though we hear that phrase all the time. It's 'carb addiction.' Those high-carbohydrate foods, the so-called 'comfort foods' are the ones you turn to when you're looking for an emotional escape."

***

In my own journey, I've found the elimination of sugar and starches is more of a social challenge than anything. Think about the calendar itself, which seems to conspire against us.

It's well known the holiday season is when we tend put on extra pounds. Part of this may be the much-maligned "Christmas Creep." It's not enough to have a couple of cookies and milk on Christmas Eve, we tuck into the candy canes and eggnog for a full month ahead of time.

But if you think about it, Christmas isn't all to blame. If we open up the definition of "holiday season" a bit, a picture starts to form. Here's a quick rundown of some of the major fall and winter holidays (religious, secular, real, and made-up). What traditional foods come to mind?

- September—"Pumpkin-Spiced Everything" season begins.
- October—Oktoberfest (along with lots of other "-fest" events centered around food, wine, etc.)
- Oct. 31—Halloween
- Early November—"Leftover Halloween Candy" season
- Late November—Thanksgiving
- December—Christmas season
- January—Football playoffs, Super Bowl Sunday
- February—Valentine's Day
- March—St. Patrick's Day
- April—Easter
- May—Cinco de Mayo

The stretch between the fall and spring equinoxes is tough for a low-carb dieter. If you think about it, we mark every special occasion by eating sugary and high-carb foods. Is it any coincidence these foods, which are shown to release the feel-good chemical dopamine in the brain, are gobbled down during the cold, dark days of winter when we are most in need of a pick-me-up?[121]

Controlling your carbohydrate intake in America today is essentially a countercultural act. We are immersed in carbs, surrounded by them. Not just at social occasions and at holiday celebrations, but on TV, radio, on our commute to work, and in the airport. (I'm pretty sure the smell alone of a Cinnabon stand contains about fifty grams of carbohydrates.)

This is where mindset becomes so important. In interviewing Dr. Cervenka and Bobbie Henry, focusing on the "big why" is a message they reinforce to their patients. "We try to get them to think of the diet as medication," Henry said. "Just as you wouldn't skip a day of epilepsy medication, for fear of having seizures, you wouldn't want to suddenly change your diet." Or, to put it more bluntly, "There are no cheat days."

This sentiment is put even more pointedly by Jade Nelson, a holistic health guide I interviewed. "There are no cheat days when it comes to brain health. If you cheat, I honestly wonder if you care enough about your wellbeing and longevity and the quality of what you can offer the people you love around you."

---

121 Robert Glatter, "The Price to Pay for Eating Highly Processed Carbohydrates," *Forbes*, June 30, 2013.

This can be a problem for patients, though, who are so immersed in the emotional, cultural, and habitual world of high-carb eating, they can't stick to the diet. Statistically, around half of the patients who try the diet quit before they have a chance to see if it works. [122]

***

Comic, voiceover professional, and podcaster Anna Vocino talks openly about the emotional side of eating, both as Vinnie Tortorich's podcast co-host and in her writing. Her cookbooks *Eat Happy* and *Eat Happy, Too,* feature "gluten-free, grain-free, low-carb recipes for a joyful life."

Even though her own journey was born out of issues with celiac disease, she spreads the message cooking and eating can still be fun and enjoyable. She tells readers, "The title of the book isn't EAT HAPPY, DAMMIT, AND THE ONLY WAY TO DO IT IS TO EAT JUST LIKE I TELL YOU TO EAT. The title is *EAT HAPPY* because I want you to figure out what you like to eat that makes you happy."[123] She adds, "I want you to retrain your brain to love eating real food, to feel full when you ARE full, and to live your life free from the bondage of diets."

Anna's journey into the low-carb lifestyle started in 2001, when her mother—after dealing with a long and painful

---

122 Fang Ye et al, "Efficacy of And Patient Compliance with a Ketogenic Diet in Adults with Intractable Epilepsy: A Meta-Analysis," *Journal of Clinical Neurology* 11 no. 1 (January 2015): 26-31.

123 Anna Vocino, *Eat Happy: Gluten Free, Grain Free, Low Carb Recipes for a Joyful Life* (Los Angeles: Telemachus Press, 2016), 18.

series of symptoms—was diagnosed with Celiac disease. She encouraged Anna to get tested too, and sure enough, it came up positive.

When she gave up gluten, she started to see improvements in small, seemingly-unrelated ways: "Immediately started to see my asthma clear up; my intestinal stuff for sure cleared up. I would still get a cold and respiratory ailments here and there, but not nearly as bad." Still, learning she could no longer eat some of her favorite foods, and eliminating those foods, was difficult. In her trademark style, Anna calls it the "temper tantrum" phase. In her best spoiled baby voice, she cries, "Wahhh! All I want is ice cream! Why can't I have it?"

"Most of us haven't figured out a way to either eat the occasional treat and be joyful about it or to just be joyful without the treat. So, we'll deprive ourselves, and then we'll have a temper tantrum that we're not 'allowed' to have it. Or we'll have the treat, but then we'll tell ourselves, 'Oh you're such a piece of shit! Why did you eat that?'" It's a struggle which illustrates just how strongly our emotions are tied to food.

Years later, Anna has managed to give up sugars, grains, and—ever since she found she was intolerant—even dairy, and it has gotten easier with time. "Though I avoid sugars and grains 95 percent of the time, I'm not a machine. I have a heart and hormones like any other lass."[124] It's a message that resonates with the millions of listeners who have downloaded her podcast over the years. "I try to be very real about what

---

124 Anna Vocino, "My Story," Anna Vocino Eat Happy, accessed October 23, 2020.

I'm going through, both when I succeed, and when I struggle," she says. "I'm very open and honest about that because we all friggin' do it; it's a universal thing."

I share with her my own Achilles' heel, beer, which has long been a hobby of mine and since college and a big part of my culture. On a diet of 20 grams of carbs or less, beer is a big no-no. (Vinnie Tortorich calls it a "glass of bread.") "Oh, man," Anna said, "So I can see you're ripe for a temper tantrum. But I'm guessing that not having a seizure is worth it."

Very true, and it has become easier over time. But like Anna, I'm not perfect; these changes don't happen overnight.

***

Mindset is also a focus of Daniel Martin who, like me, found the diet-epilepsy connection quite by accident. I met Daniel through Facebook, and he was eager to share his story. Even through the distance of Zoom, his energy and enthusiasm seemed to radiate from the screen.

As a computer programmer in his twenties, he found his weight creeping up on him and wanted to do something about it. "Some crazy neighbors of mine were doing this thing called *Whole 30*," a diet that cuts out grains, dairy, preservatives and other foods. Even though he did it for weight loss, he found that for the first time, "I made the connection between what you eat and how you look and how you feel."

The experience motivated him to explore further, and he eventually found keto. He found the diet easy and delicious, but it also made him feel empowered. "I wasn't even doing it for epilepsy at this point," he says, "but I started to realize I had some control over every speck of acne, every strand of hair, every neuron, how happy or depressed or anxious I feel. I started to see that I can fix these different things."

He began to wonder what else he could control through diet. "I looked at my epilepsy medication and I'm like, 'Dude, I don't know. I've been lucky to be controlled by this for so long. But there's no guarantees, right?' I want to take power into my own hands instead of being a prisoner of the medication system, of the doctor, and of being worried I'll have a seizure all the time."

"I thought, well, I'm already doing the diet designed for epilepsy, so I made it my goal to be healthy enough that I don't have seizures anymore."

Like Jennifer, he weaned himself off of medication and carefully tracked his diet instead. The transition was a struggle—he had several seizures while trying to adjust and optimize his diet—but to him it was worth it. "I felt normal. I felt good. I felt happy. I felt like I'm more in tune with my mind and in tune with my body."

One of the keys to the whole experience, he says, is mindset. "I like to use that word because it's kind of all-encompassing. Encompassing of positive thinking, meditation, spirituality, relaxation, anti-stress...all these things together. You're never in complete control of your external environment; a plane could crash, you could wake up with cancer or some terrible thing, but you're always in control of how you respond to anything."

Again, I don't recommend going it alone the way that Daniel has. As empowering as it is to take control of one's own health, the guidance of a knowledgable practitioner is the best way to optimize powerful interventions like medication and lifestyle.

***

Meeting Anna and Daniel on successive days was like finding the yin and yang of healthy mindset. It was about letting go of the emotional ties to food and embracing a way forward—changing the negative, deprivation-based thoughts to more positive, heath-focused ones.

I must admit there are still struggles. Food is, as Cywes says, not just nutrition. It's celebration, connection, comfort, and escape. I'm learning to divert those cravings to lower-carb alternatives—trading chips and dip for salami and cheese, for example—but two years in, it's still a process. Habits and emotions are formidable foes for any mindset. One thing that seems to help, though, is finding what many writers call a "big why." In other words, connecting these habits to a larger purpose.

CHAPTER 13

EATING FOR LIFE: THE POWER OF PURPOSE

When Charlie Abrahams became seizure-free, Jim and Nancy dedicated their time and resources to spreading the word. The Charlie Foundation became the preeminent voice of ketogenic diet therapy and, thanks to their efforts, the diet has survived and is a success today.

They are an example of how something as simple as a way of eating can become something much larger: a vision or a mission. In fact, there are many who have found in this diet not just a new lease on life, but a new livelihood.

***

Lean, handsome, and energetic, ivy-league educated Krishna Kaliannan is the very picture of the twenty-first-century entrepreneur. His company Catalina Crunch exploded from an idea of making low-carb cereal in his kitchen to doing over a million dollars a month in direct-to-consumer sales, and it has the kind of loyal following many companies dream of. But the inspiration for his company goes all the way back to a high-school diagnosis of epilepsy.

I spoke to Krishna on the phone one evening right at the start of the COVID-19 pandemic. He was in his New York City apartment, and I could hear a big ruckus going on in the background. It was the city's residents applauding the first responders from their windows. We both have reason to be thankful for their work.

"I didn't know it at the time, but I had my first seizure the during the summer after my junior year in high school." It was his first night of a summer program at University of Pennsylvania, where he'd eventually go to school. "I'd just gotten into Philly for a couple months of classes at Penn, and I was really excited—real nervous as well, obviously." After a long, sleepless night in the dorm room, he had his first seizure. "Thing is, I didn't know it was a seizure at the time. My mind went blank and I woke up a couple of hours later. I was lying on the ground, my head hurt, and I was confused. But I'm not sure I even knew what epilepsy and seizures were at the time. I thought I'd just fallen asleep."

He became angry with himself for oversleeping. "I dressed quickly, and looking back, I realize that I'd put everything on backward. It was crazy. I actually managed to put my dress shoes on the wrong feet. I put my shirt on inside out. So, I sprinted off to the office to find out where classes are held, and the lady there, she's looking at me like I'm crazy."

He eventually made it to class and struggled through the rest of the day. It would be almost another year, though, before he'd realize he'd had a seizure.

This time, he was at home. His mother called 911, and he was rushed to the hospital. A visit to a neurologist, who did an EEG, confirmed he had epilepsy. "Once I had that seizure, I sort of realized the first experience had also been a seizure."

***

One thing that frustrated Krishna about life with a diagnosis, though, was being tied to medication. "What drove me crazy is how they give you a thirty-day supply, which meant I had to go back to the pharmacy every thirty days. And the stuff wasn't cheap, either."

When he got to college, he carried with him a six-month supply of his medication. "So, you know, you have six months until you need to go back and see the doctor," which, to a college freshman getting settled into a new life, seems like a long way off—but not all that far. "I'm a freshman in college, it's the six-month mark, and all of a sudden CVS was going, 'Hey we can't give you any more epilepsy medication because your prescription is out of date.' I got so angry about that. This medication is my lifeline."

After "throwing a fit at CVS" and getting nowhere, it took him several days to find a neurologist who could see him and get him a new prescription. In the meantime he had his third seizure, this time in the dorm's shower. "It was kind of embarrassing," he admits. "Here's the ambulance, coming into the middle of the public dorm to drag me back to the hospital."

His university's hospital was a research hospital, and as it happened the neurologist there was starting a study on the ketogenic diet. "I was one of the first people in that study," he said. The doctors advised him to restrict his carbohydrates to 20 grams per day and to track everything in a journal for six months, which, for a college freshman, is a tall order. "Here I was in Philly, looking forward to eating Philly cheesesteaks, but that kind of went out the window."

After six months he was also able to gradually back off his epilepsy medication, Keppra, from 3000 mg to 1000 mg per day, a dose he still takes. The benefit was not just financial; one of the side effects of Keppra is its tendency to make people quick to anger. "Keppra rage" is a term that is well-known in the epilepsy community. "I didn't notice it, but my mom did feel I was more prone to getting angry. Once I looked into it, I realized scientists don't know exactly how this drug works. They just know it has an overall dulling effect on the brain, which tends to reduce the chance you have a seizure. So, I wasn't super-excited about taking this stuff." Using diet alongside this lower dose, he's had only two seizures in the ten years since then, both when he's forgotten to take the medication.

***

As with many others, there was a kind of serendipity at play here. Krishna found this diet because he visited the research doctor who was conducting the study. Not everyone is so lucky. But one difference from then to now is the availability of information through the internet. "Back in the day, to learn about any of this stuff you had to go to a medical university and get your MD then go practice and learn from others, but now obviously with Google Scholar and just the internet in general, you have all sorts of folks who can just learn and get quite far on their own."

This do-it-yourself attitude translates to a positive outlook on living with his diagnosis. "It is what you make of it. You know, you can wallow around in sadness forever over the fact that it's a part of your life, or you can try to do something about it." This attitude took Krishna into the next phase of his life.

Ten years after the fateful six-month study at Penn, Krishna was eating breakfast with his girlfriend one morning. "On this research experiment, it was eggs all the time. Just eggs, eggs, eggs, and more eggs. Now here I am ten years later, and I was so sick of eggs I would have eaten anything else." He'd spent many mornings watching his girlfriend enjoy waffles, French toast, and all manner of high-carb breakfast goodies.

His frustration gave birth to a whole new idea: a low-carb cereal. "I grew up with Cocoa Puffs, Waffle Crisp, and Cinnamon Toast Crunch, and I missed that stuff." So, he started experimenting in his kitchen. "My first attempt tasted awful," he laughs. "I figured, 'Cacao, that's just like chocolate, right?' But I didn't realize at the time cacao is really bitter, that they add a lot of milk and sugar to make it palatable." He continued to experiment and eventually came up with a recipe for an almond-flour-based cereal both low-carb and delicious.

His hobby became a career when a friend of his, who was trying the keto diet, asked to try some. The friend liked it and, unsolicited, sent Krishna a payment for it through Venmo. "And then before I knew it, you know, he was wanting some every week, and then one of his friends wanted some every week; all of a sudden there was like ten or twelve people who all wanted me to bake cereal for them. It kind of became 'a thing.'"

That "thing" is now Catalina Crunch, and within a year it was generating almost a million dollars a month in sales.

Krishna's is an incredible success story—not just of managing epilepsy, but of finding a career and a calling. He believes deeply the food we put in your body matters and eating keto should not be difficult or painful. When I asked him about his company's mission, he said, "We are really out to prove to the world that eating keto or eating low carb can taste delicious."

He's not the only one who has built the ketogenic diet into a lifestyle, and that lifestyle into a livelihood. Engineer Michel Lundell, inventor of the Ketonix breath ketone analyzer, is another person who turned epilepsy and ketosis into a life purpose. What is it about the ketogenic lifestyle that turns patients into converts of such fervor? I sat down with him to find out.

***

Like me, Lundell, an engineer in Sweden, was diagnosed with epilepsy as an adult. He had his first grand mal seizure in

2004. "My wife didn't know it was a grand mal. She thought I was going to die or something," he says. At first, doctors misdiagnosed the cause as a brain tumor. "They saw something on my brain scan, and that was a wake-up call."

But after six months and several more tests, the doctors determined it wasn't a tumor after all, and perhaps the seizure was nothing to worry about. "They said, 'Well, it's probably just one seizure. Anybody can have a seizure,'" he says. But six years later, he had another grand mal, this time while driving with his family. He woke up in the hospital and came out with a prescription.

At first, it was fine. "At a very low dose of this medication, I found I had a mental clarity. I could focus very easily on things." But as doctors doubled the dose and doubled it again—eventually up to a tenfold increase—to reach the right blood levels, "I got more and more screwed up in my head. I became this sort of angry person. My wife and my kids noticed; I mean the kids couldn't be kids anymore. I would yell at them to be quiet when they were playing in the house, that sort of thing." His wife gave him an ultimatum: change or move out.

He began looking for alternatives to medication and found the ketogenic diet. "It worked with kids who were having ten seizures a day. Mine wasn't so bad, so I thought it should work for me." He told his neurologist he wanted to try it. "He said, 'I have to look into this.' He actually didn't know about it, himself." His doctor was open to it, though, and willing to find out more. "He went away for two weeks, and he came back with a big pile of papers from all the way back to the

Bible to recent studies. It turned out he had some colleagues who were doing studies on this, and they said in some ways it was even better than drugs."

His doctor had concerns about the difficulty of the diet and about compliance, but he agreed to try it if Lundell could come back a month later and show that he was in ketosis. The strange thing was, Lundell said, "They couldn't tell me what level of ketosis I had to be in. I wanted to measure something."

There are two common methods of measuring ketones: in the urine or in the blood (in other words, peeing on a strip or poking your finger). Lundell tried both. "I was confused, because one day the numbers would come up high in the blood, but low on the pee strip, and the next day vice versa. I was scratching my head and asking myself, how could this be?" Nevertheless, his neurologist was satisfied with Lundell's test results and agreed to help phase out the drugs.

***

Being an engineer, Lundell set his mind to figuring out the best way to measure ketosis. "We engineers solve problems all day; that's what we do. It's what triggers us. If I didn't have this, I'd solve puzzles or something."

It turns out urine strips, which measure a ketone called acetyl acetate, are known to have several issues in terms of reliability. For one thing, the level can be influenced by how hydrated or dehydrated you are and how diluted the ketones become. For another, ketones in the urine are in some ways "extra." You're peeing them out because your body doesn't need them.[125]

The finger prick, which measures a chemical called beta-hydroxybutyrate, is known to be better, but it also isn't perfect. "Blood ketones are formed when ketosis actually goes down," Lundell said. The acetyl acetate is packed into a stable molecule in the blood called beta-hydroxybutyrate, so it can be used later. "It's a storage mechanism. The cells create blood ketones and put them into the bloodstream. Your liver gets the signal and says, 'I don't need to make as many ketones anymore.'"

"If you just sit and eat a lot of fat bombs, for example, you will get a high number of blood ketones. So, you might say, 'Oh, now I'm burning fat.' But this doesn't mean you're actually more in ketosis." There's one other problem with measuring blood ketones: the strips are expensive, costing up to a dollar each.

The best way to measure whether ketones were being produced, Lundell realized, would be to go to the source: the liver. In the process of ketogenesis, the liver does all the work of turning fat into ketones; but what's the best way to measure that directly? The research indicated acetone, sometimes called an "exhaust" ketone because it's emitted in the breath every time the liver produces ketones, held the key. "When there is any breakdown of fat into ketone energy, breath ketones are released."

---

125 "Advantages Using Ketonix," Ketonix Breath Ketone Analyzer, accessed October 25, 2020.

"I wondered if acetone was something you could measure," he says. "Other researchers had tried it," and found it to be accurate, "but the available machines were very, very expensive. I wanted something simple you could use before breakfast, after breakfast, before training and after training...a tool to help you to learn how your body reacts to certain foods and exercise, so you could create a lifestyle that would keep you in ketosis. I just wanted to know is one egg good, two eggs? Is coconut oil good for me? How much protein could I eat in one day and stay in ketosis? In blood and urine ketones, you don't get that response."

Lundell created what's now known as the Ketonix, a portable, easy-to-use device that measures breath ketones. It's about the size of a pen, with a valve on one end and a light-up display on the side. It has many advantages over the other tests. Instead of peeing on a plastic strip or poking your finger with a lancet, you simply blow into the valve. Instead of trying to judge the color of a pee-strip or reading the numbers on a digital display, you watch as a light turns yellow, green, blue, or red to indicate how many ketones you're producing. With no disposable strips or lancets, the device—which can be used thousands of times—makes for an economical and eco-friendly long-term choice.

The Ketonix now ships all over the world, and Lundell speaks at conferences and in forums teaching doctors, researchers, and laypeople about the ins and outs of ketosis and breath ketone measuring.

As we talk, Lundell shows me his latest innovation, a Ketonix app. It will allow users to store their ketone readings long-term, track their diet, exercise, and more so they can figure out the causal relationship between their lifestyle choices and their ketone levels. His enthusiasm is infectious, and I can't wait to get my hands on one. It's clear to me his mission is not just to solve this puzzle of measuring ketosis and lifestyle, but to help others to find their own best ketogenic life. Thanks to his device, he says, "It has never been easier to create a healthy lifestyle."

***

Speaking with Krishna and Lundell, I am reminded it's not just about adopting a lifestyle; it's about creating a life. Both men have found more than just health in the ketogenic lifestyle. They've found purpose. They've also helped countless others to better their lives. They're wonderful examples of how food and lifestyle can connect us to something larger in the world.

Whether it's through starting companies, working with patients or clients, or speaking at conferences or on a podcast, there are now many people who have turned this lifestyle into a life—so many it's become a sort of community enabled through the internet and social media. This is important because if there's any aspect of lifestyle change too often overlooked, it's community.

CHAPTER 14

DIET TRIBES: THE POWER OF COMMUNITY

—

I have a real love-hate relationship with social media. A typical weekend for me starts with posting a photo of my dogs Jake and Buddy on a morning hike and ends with firing my phone across the bedroom, cursing it for keeping me up too late on a Sunday night. I'm always the last person I know to create a Twitter/Instagram/TikTok/Whatever-the-Next-Thing-Is account, and I've canceled my Facebook account several times over the years.

I was on the verge of dropping out again when I heard Vinnie Tortorich talk on his podcast about the NSNG Facebook group. He said it was a group he didn't create and doesn't manage, but it does have his name on it. Curious, I took my finger off the "delete" button and signed up.

The group, now with close to twenty-seven thousand members, is an active, buzzing place. It includes fans of the podcast and of Vinnie's book and movie. Veteran group members, sharing Vinnie's irreverent sense of humor, give out advice and good-natured ribbing to newbies and share their own before-and-after photos, labeled with such themes as "Transformation Tuesday" and "Facelift Friday"(although "Topless Thursday" was discontinued when things got a little out-of-hand). Facebook quickly became "NSNGbook" for me as the community turned into my go-to for questions, inspiration, and a few laughs.

Meagan North-Hawkes is one of several administrators of the group. I reached out to her to ask about her own NSNG journey. "I started in December 2017, a couple of days before Christmas. I had gotten my physical and they called me the next day and said I had diabetes. Me being who I am, I'm like, 'No, I don't! I mean, yes, okay I may be obese, but...' Looking back, I don't know how I could think I didn't have it. But I took it to heart, and I gave up sugar that day."

At her follow-up appointment two weeks later, she had lost seven pounds. She told her doctor she wanted to continue, and he agreed to hold off on medication. "I'd watched my mom give herself insulin shots my whole life, and I knew I didn't want to do that." Meagan continued visiting for follow-up appointments every few months, and over the course of the next two years, her blood sugar, A1C, blood pressure, and cholesterol normalized. She also lost one hundred and twenty-five pounds.

I asked Meagan how the Facebook group played into her amazing success. "I joined the group pretty early on. I've always been a person who wants to do it all on my own. I'm not going to ask for help; I'm just going to do it. I set my mind, and then that's kind of it. But I realized quickly that with such a big change, you can't. This is bigger than anything I've ever done before."

She began to build a team to help her get there, including a trainer and a life coach. "We all have strengths and weaknesses," she says. "You need someone to point out to you when you're falling into thinking habits that aren't helpful. You need a tribe."

Having a tribe or a team is important, too, to overcome the barriers isolation can raise. "I feel like most people who are obese kind of lose who they are. For me, I withdrew more, I didn't want to go out, and I didn't want to be with my friends. But in the process of losing the weight, I gained confidence, and I feel like I became the person I was when I was younger, that person that I forgot I was."

Meagan's words really spoke to me. I tend to be a do-it-yourselfer, sometimes to a fault. My thinking goes: I *created* this problem by myself, I should be able to *solve* this problem by myself. But I've begun to recognize this as a trap.

It's a balancing act, finding ways to take responsibility for your health, but at the same time recognizing when you need help and asking for it. You might think, of all people, the guy who spent a year bumming rides off his friends and had to be rescued from a hospital somewhere would know this better than anyone else and would be intimately familiar with the power of interdependence. But it's still a struggle and still a lesson I have to learn again and again.

***

The power of support is clear in many of the people I've spoken to. For Gillian Szollos, it was her husband who found the ketogenic diet (again, through a Facebook community) and her husband who helped her to stay on it. For me, my wife Judy is my support; she has now joined me in doing away with the rice and the high-carb treats so as to help keep me on the path.

My friend Shila is another great example of this power. When she went on a ketogenic diet to lose weight, she got the whole family on board. "Initially, it was hard because I had to make two types of food every day." The traditional Persian recipes her two young sons were used often included bread or rice. By searching online, she found low-carb substitutes for many of their favorites.

Getting the kids involved in the process, she says, was key to winning them over: "They love cooking and helping out— making salads, roasting vegetables." The boys picked up on her healthy habits, too. "When we go grocery shopping, they read the back to see the sugar levels and the carbohydrate level. It's gotten to the point that if I mistakenly pick up something high in carbs, they'll correct me," she laughs. "It's good because they're educating themselves and they're making better decisions. It's become a teaching tool.

***

Support is particularly important when the lifestyle you're trying to adopt runs counter to the culture you're in. According to Kelly McGonigal, PhD and author of *The Willpower Instinct*, "Humans are hard-wired to connect with others." In order to ensure this connection, specialized brain cells called "mirror neurons" cause us to unconsciously mimic what people around us are doing. According to McGonigal, "Our instinct to mirror other people's actions means that when you see someone reach for a snack, a drink, or a credit card, you may find yourself unconsciously mirroring their behavior."[126]

This is because "trusting the judgment of others is the glue that makes social living work." It's what ensures acceptance by and membership in our communities.

The good news is this effect can work in our favor, too. McGonigal describes a study in Tennessee in which church leaders pointed their congregation to biblical passages discouraging excessive eating and drinking and encouraging care for one's physical health. They were able to get parishioners to adopt healthy habits by connecting with their existing values, as well as leveraging their community membership. According to McGonigal, "We may be willing to give up our vices and cultivate new virtues if we believe it will more firmly secure a spot in our most cherished tribe."[127]

---

126 Kelly McGonigal, *The Willpower Instinct: How Self-Control Works, Why it Matters, and What You Can Do to Get More of It*, (New York: Avery, 2012):188.

127 Ibid., 197-198.

***

The NSNG group is one of many low-carb-oriented groups on Facebook. Once I started going down the rabbit hole, I found groups about keto recipes, keto athletics, keto lifestyle, and even one about the ketogenic diet and epilepsy. This is how I first met Dr. Inna Hughes, who I introduced earlier.

When Dr. Hughes started working closely with the registered dietitian at the University of Rochester hospital, she learned of a gap in the system: a neurologist would identify children who are candidates for the ketogenic diet, then pass them off to the dietician. "The dietician would go, 'Okay, now what do I do?'" She would start the patients on the diet, but her role as an RD meant she was limited in the ways she could work with the patient—more so than the referring neurologist might have realized. "I'm a nosy do-gooder," Dr. Hughes jokes, "so I made it my mission to fix this system."

She and the dietician started meeting with the patients together. In doing so, "we could look at the patient's biology, their development, and their nutrition all together, along with the management of their epilepsy and management of their meds."

This bigger-picture view of each patient has another advantage: "You can start to see there are trends. So, there's a clear trend that people can absorb their medication differently before the diet and after the diet. There is a clear trend that we need to keep on top of growth patterns for kids. As you collect these patient experiences, you start to see trends and patterns."

For Dr. Hughes, the simple tweak of teaming up and working closely with an RD has allowed her to understand each patient better—the particular jumble of interrelations happening within each part of the human body and brain—but also to advance the research and our understanding of the ways that the ketogenic diet works as a whole.

Nor is this simply academic. She's able to share insights and takeaways with her patients through Facebook. She helps to run a private group called "The Ketogenic Diet and Epilepsy," which started as a support group for local families but now has more than eight hundred people from around the world. "It has been tremendously useful in treatment," she says. "We get everything in the group from, 'Been there, done that, got the t-shirt' to, 'What the hell is happening and where do we start?' If we can connect those families that are just starting out to those who have already been through it, they can share ideas, and they can help each other to get through this very difficult emotional experience."

The fact Dr. Hughes, with her knowledge, positivity, and genuine excitement for the mission of helping her patients, participates in and moderates the group gives it a professionalism and positivity rarely found in online communities. People there are supportive, giving, and sincere. In short, it works.

Epilepsy is a lonely disorder. It is more common than you might think, sure, but it's easy to feel you're the only one dealing with this terrifying thing. Add to that the challenge of upending your dietary patterns and sometimes your entire lifestyle, and it's easy to see why many families struggle. By creating a community of support, Dr. Hughes has essentially created wraparound services and ongoing intervention for her patients, so even when they're not in the office, they don't have to feel like they're in out the wilderness.

***

There is something powerful here. Chronic diseases can be healed with chronic therapies—not just pharmaceuticals and devices—but it falls to the patient to comply. The American Diabetes Association recently acknowledged low-carb diets can be effective in treating the disease which affects nearly 11 percent of Americans.[128] But here's the rub: it's much easier to take a pill once a day than it is to change one's diet at every meal. Motivation flags, challenges arise. Dr. Hughes's Facebook group helps patients to recharge their motivation, supporting one another through those challenges. By leveraging the power of social media, she's created a "tribe" of her own, allowing for better mental health for stressed out parents and physical and neurological health for their children.

128 Adele Hite, "American Diabetes Association Endorses Low-Carb Diet as Option," Diet Doctor, April 25, 2019.

CHAPTER 15

SACRED DISEASES: THE POWER OF DEFINING YOURSELF

———

In his book *Atomic Habits*, James Clear gives readers a useful framework for thinking about goal setting and habit change. The first layer, he says, is about outcomes. "I want to lose weight" is an example of an outcome-based goal. The second layer is processes, goals that center on the things you want to do such as going to the gym every day, rather than the outcome you want to see. The third and, Clear says, deepest layer is about identity. An identity-based goal is about not just the *what* or the *how*, but the *who*—who you want to be. In other words, "I want to be a healthy person." Clear says, "Outcomes are about what you get. Processes are about what you do. Identity is about what you believe." [129]

———

129 James Clear, *Atomic Habits: An Easy & Proven Way to Build Good Habits & Break Bad Ones,* Read by the author (New York: Penguin Audio, 2018), Audible audio ed., 5hrs, 25 min.

His advice for anyone hoping to make a change—whether it be in your diet, your career, or any other aspect of life—is simple: "1. Decide the type of person you want to be. 2. Prove it to yourself with small wins." The small actions we take every day (like going to the gym) reinforce our self-image as the kind of person we want to be (a person who cares about health).

Dr. Robert Cywes has some controversial insights about how food and identity intertwine. "Why is it 98 percent of ketogenic diets are going to fail? And yet most vegans can sustain a vegan way of life for an extremely long time?" The difference, he says, is most people take up a ketogenic diet as a short-term solution to a problem—losing weight, lowering blood sugar, etc.—so in Clear's language, people take it up with an outcome-based goal. "So, when somebody on a ketogenic diet is offered a piece of cake, the typical response is, 'Oh, no, no, no, I'm not allowed to have that. I'm on a keto diet.' It sounds like deprivation."[130]

On the other hand, Cywes points out, if you offer steak to a vegetarian or vegan animal-rights lover, "They don't say, 'Oh no, I'm not allowed to eat that.' They say, 'Damn you, you killed Bambi!'" Cywes calls this perspective "arrogant integrity." In other words, the person has embraced an identity as an animal-rights-loving vegetarian and the beliefs and values going along with it. The "arrogance" of being someone who doesn't eat meat—and believing not doing so forms the basis for their identity—leads to "integrity" in sticking to this way of eating.

---

130 Robert Cywes, "Arrogant Integrity," Facebook video, February 19, 2020.

His suggestion for people attempting a ketogenic lifestyle is to adopt the same kind of arrogant integrity. Instead of seeing carbohydrates as something you're missing out on, see it as something you wouldn't touch—cheap, addictive, low-quality filler foods existing only to hijack the brain and harm the body.

This might sound extreme, but it's been a tremendous help to me in my own journey. It's easier to skip the breadsticks before dinner when you realize they're only there to stimulate a hormonal response in the body, making you order more food. It's easier to skip the bun on the burger when you realize it's just there to make the meat more palatable. (Try a plain Mickey D's patty sometime, and you'll see what I mean.) Actions like these reinforce my identity as someone who cares about food—good food—and who also cares about my health. It's an important shift for many reasons, particularly as someone who is still learning to live with a diagnosis.

***

What is it to live with a diagnosis? To be a person with a diagnosis? A diagnosis is a powerful thing. It's concrete. It's one of those rare things we all search for in life: an answer. That thing that went click in your knee? That pain in your back? That tightness, that kink, that owie? It's a question, an effect that wants a cause. Once we get that cause, then we can get rid of the pain. So, we seek the comfort of a diagnosis.

The problem with a diagnosis is it can become *too* powerful. It can start to become an identity. A person with epilepsy becomes an "epileptic." This can be a slippery slope. When we talk about ways to manage it, then we are really talking about ways to define ourselves.

Jade Nelson is a massage therapist and holistic health guide. She works with clients both locally and internationally to offer nutrition information, yoga, massage, self-care consults, mindset coaching, and more. She describes herself as "a Pandora's magical box of health and wellness knowledge."

"I walk the path of the wounded healer," she says, invoking a kind of shamanistic language of transcending the physical into the realm of the spiritual. This is the presence she brings to our interview; I can see at once she is a wise, down-to-earth, thoughtful person who cares and feels deeply.

Jade had her first seizure at seven years old and was diagnosed with epilepsy at the age of eight. "'The train inside me' was how I described it as a child when a seizure was coming. I always had about a ten-minute aura or warning; I could feel it coming. I heard the sound of a very loud, like a train coming down the track. I could hear it in the distance. That's what I heard in my head when a seizure was coming, and it would just barrel at you. That's what it felt like. As it got closer, it would literally feel like it was running over my body, like you were being run over by a train."[131]

Speaking at KetoCon, she rattles off the shocking statistics of her youth: three ICU stays, twelve EEGs, seventeen MRIs all before the age of eighteen, and thirty complex-partial

---

131 Jimmy Moore, "1359: Jade Nelson Finds the Train Inside of Her with Keto Epilepsy Journey," January 30, 2018, in *The Livin' La Vida Low Carb Show*, podcast, MP3 audio, 40:07.

seizures she can remember. "The hospital was my second home," she states.[132]

Over the years she tried ten different medications, with varying levels of success. "I'd gone up to four years seizure-free, but always with lots of side-effects." At the time she discovered keto, she was on Zanicimide and was struggling. "I'd lost over twenty pounds—I was extremely underweight—and I had gastritis." After about a year of this, her sister called. "I basically got a call from my sister who said 'Have you thought about the ketogenic diet? I know you'd have to change a lot, since you don't eat dairy, and you don't eat pork or beef...' I said I thought it was only for pediatrics, but that was not the case."

She grew up with a mother who is a nurse and a family focused on health. "We were the weird family on the block that ate the weird food," she jokes. So, it wasn't a complete surprise that food might help treat her epilepsy. She set to work doing her research.

"I'd been loosely paleo for a while, but I still liked to eat a lot of sugar—coconut sugar and things like that." When her sister came to her with this information, she says, "I was all in. It only took me two days to make up my mind, and I never looked back."

Two days later, she called her doctor and asked him to take her off of her medication. The doctor said "Great, I support

---

132 Jade Nelson, "Epilepsy & Keto: My Journey of Healing in the Kitchen," Keto Con 2018, July 16, 2018, YouTube Video, 37:45.

you doing that." Although he didn't have the background to help her, he was able to point her to the resources at the Charlie Foundation website.

She settled on a diet of no more than 50 grams of carbohydrates a day. Her family was very supportive as she made the transition to this whole new way of eating, but others weren't so sure. "I've had people say I was going to ruin my health eating this way. My doctor was supportive as best as he could, but he couldn't really provide me with much help."

She did have her struggles at the start. "I would be lying if I didn't say it wasn't hard in the beginning. It was trying to find that balance of how to be out in public, how to order food at a restaurant, how to make it look like nothing is different, but also being able to say, 'I'm on a medical diet.'"

***

The diet was not a miracle cure, but it did allow her to cut back on the medications that were so expensive and were affecting her life. "I had no idea how much it would change my life. I'm on the least amount of meds I've ever been on. All I can say is I'm actually content for the first time in my life. I feel hopeful. I feel empowered now because of this diet, and I have learned so much information I just want to share it with other people."

On the other hand, Jade says, "I don't want people to think the ketogenic diet is going to fix everything, because I went four years on the ketogenic diet without having seizures and then I had two. The reality is, some of us will be lucky and will be able to go seizure free, but not all." She says she doesn't believe in "cures," but she does believe in management of epilepsy and of healing for the brain.

It's an important reminder. "Epilepsy is impacted by many different things. It's not just the food we eat. It's whether we sleep well enough, our stress levels, the environment, the weather." The diet has altered her life, she says, but more importantly, it's altered her perspective on wellness and health. "It's simply become how I live. I don't even think twice anymore about what needs to be cooked, how to eat something, or whether it needs to be measured properly."

Another aspect she emphasizes is food sensitivities. Some high-fat and low-carb foods can still cause trouble. Cheese is a big culprit for many of her clients. They may be doing everything right, but they find their ketones are still low. For many of these people cutting down on dairy, and cheese in particular, can be exactly what they need.

***

At the end of our interview, Jade's healer instinct seems to kick in and she flips the interview around on me. She asks, "When you think about epilepsy, do you see it as a chronic illness, a disorder, or a disease?"

The question catches me off guard—embarrassingly so. I'm a writer, after all, and I believe words matter. Yet I've heard—and probably used—these terms interchangeably over the years without giving it much thought. "You need to figure it out," she says, smiling, "otherwise you can't use my story."

I am caught flat-footed. I stammer around the question a bit. This, I realize, gets to the heart of why I'm writing this book. How I view my diagnosis is, in some respects, how I view myself. Am I a functioning human? A capable adult? Or am I somehow something less? An adult with an asterisk at the end?

She finally let me off the hook and gives me her view. As she does, her eyes light up and her voice grows stronger. The passion she brings to her life and her work—if they can even be separated—is clear. "Technically epilepsy is a disorder; it's not a disease." Diseases can be cured, she says, while epilepsy can be managed. "Whether someone wants to call it a chronic illness? That's a personal choice, I suppose. But I don't want to be labeled that way. Ever."

I tell her a story of my own. A few days after my last seizure at work, I was talking to a woman in our HR department about some paperwork. She told me she was sorry to hear about what happened and offered whatever help I needed. "I'm also in charge of disability accommodations," she said, "so...in case you need anything there." I felt the phone receiver tingle in my hand. Disability? As in, disabled? Me? It's a label I don't want to self-apply.

Jade agrees. "I've seen over the years how the medical field has evolved and how people with diagnoses end up choosing to use them as a crutch or an excuse for why they can't be functioning humans or learning how to work within their means and what they're capable of." As for her, she says, "Each time I had a seizure, I had a choice to give up or put myself back together. I choose the latter over and over again."[133]

I love the way she reframes epilepsy: "It's something that happens to me, but it's not who I am." So often, we look for the easy way to define people—the name tag to pin on someone. You're a teacher. You're an executive. You're a parent. You're a yuppie. It's our need to save precious mental space by reducing everything to easy categories. Fighting it is futile. The problem, though, comes when we pin these labels on ourselves. Epilepsy is part of my life, but not all of my life. In writing this book, am I slapping on that name tag? I wonder.

But what's the other option? Keep this part of me hidden? In the end, my choice is to tell the story or not. I can only hope in telling it I can help others to understand.

When Hippocrates called epilepsy "The Sacred Disease," he meant it ironically. In his writings, he argued *against* the idea seizures were caused by possession of spirits good or evil and advanced the position it could be treated with medical, rather than spiritual, cures.

In speaking to Jade Nelson and hearing her perspective as a healer, it strikes me perhaps she's found a middle path between these opposing ideas. By using nutrition, movement, and self-care, she's developed a larger perspective—one not hiding from her diagnosis, but one not dominated by it either. Instead, she focuses on the path forward to healing

---

133 Jade Nelson, "Meet Jade," Jade Jelson: Hope, Strength, and Wisdom, accessed October 23, 2020.

and strength. As she states on her website, "I refer to my diagnosis as a 'gift.' A gift in lessons of healing that has allowed me to shape a magical mindset, which has given me the ability to flow through adversity with understanding and acceptance."[134]

---

134 Ibid.

CHAPTER 16

THE FUTURE OF FAT: THE POWER OF KNOWLEDGE

—————

So, somehow I, with my unremarkable brain, managed to stumble onto a weight-loss diet which also helps with epilepsy, or an epilepsy diet also helping people lose weight. I found some principles to help me stick with it. But the thing that helped the most—helped cement my purpose, my resolve, and my mindset—was continuing to learn.

As the months went on, I filled my morning commute with keto and low-carb podcasts, followed researchers and practitioners on Twitter, and even signed up for virtual conferences when I found them. I was slowly being drawn into the world of keto-mania.

The more I listened, the more I heard about effects beyond weight and epilepsy. Bloggers and podcast interviewees would talk about how a low-carb diet helped with their migraines, psychological issues, IBS, fibromyalgia, polycystic ovarian syndrome, autism, Alzheimer's, Parkinson's, and even cancer—impressive side-effects for a weight-loss fad. As a healthy skeptic, I began to grow suspicious. Perhaps this was one of those man-with-a-hammer situations where everything looked like a nail, or perhaps I'd stumbled upon the twenty-first-century version of Bernarr Macfadden's health cult. It was starting to sound like a snake-oil sales pitch, like a Magic Bullet.

***

Jong Rho, MD, chief of pediatric neurology at University of California, San Diego and the Rady Children's Hospital, shed some light on the question during his talk at this year's Metabolic Health Summit. In his presentation, he shared a slide—adapted from Dr. Kossoff's work—featuring a list of no less than twenty-six disorders that have been or are currently being studied by researchers as applications of the ketogenic diet and noted "this list is actually growing."[135] How can one little change, like cutting carbs, treat so many different conditions?

According to Dr. Rho, "metabolism-based treatments, typified by the ketogenic diet, are like a magic shotgun, not a magic bullet." It's not a one-size-fits-all, but it is one up-front change that has many downstream effects. Or in science-speak, "there are a lot of different targets and pathways

---

135 John Rho, MD, "Diet and the Brain: Is There a Bona Fide Scientific Connection?" PowerPoint presentation, Metabolic Health Summit, Long Beach CA, January 30, 2020.

that are affected" by the ketogenic diet.[136] His talk presents the latest research showing that the diet affects the way the brain creates energy through cell metabolism, regulates levels of different neurotransmitters like adenosine, reduces inflammation—not just in the brain but throughout the body—reduces free radicals in the body, and changes the makeup of the gut microbiome. A powerful shotgun, indeed.

***

I spoke with Dr. Susan Masino, PhD, the Vernon D. Roosa Professor of Applied Science at Trinity College, who has a joint appointment in neuroscience and psychology. She's the editor of the text *Ketogenic Diet and Metabolic Therapies: Expanded Roles in Health and Disease,* which was way over my head but gives a comprehensive overview of the many applications of the ketogenic diet. Dr. Masino spent years studying the connection between ketosis and adenosine, but she tells me it is this very multifaceted nature of the diet that makes it difficult to study.[137]

"I think the diet's superpower, which is also its Achilles' heel when you go to grant reviews, is that it works via multiple mechanisms. And the problem with science and grant reviews is they want to know, 'What is the mechanism?' It's supposed to be the National Institute of Health, but it's really sometimes like the National Institute of What's the

---

136 Ibid.

137 Susan Masino et al, "Adenosine, Ketogenic Diet and Epilepsy: The Emerging Therapeutic Relationship Between Metabolism and Brain Activity," *Current Neuropharmacology* 7, no. 3 (March 2009): 257-68.

Mechanism? That may have impeded opportunities to test metabolic therapies."

This may be changing, given the number of ketogenic diet studies published recently and currently underway. PubMed, a website run by the NIH, allows anyone and everyone to easily search the world's largest database of medical publications. Type in "ketogenic," and you'll get over four thousand results.[138] What's interesting is the bar graph in the upper-left-hand corner of the page plots the results by year; the slope is flat from 1927 to about 2000, when it starts to rocket upward. So far this year, four hundred and fifty-five new articles have been published. Meanwhile, a quick search of the term "ketogenic" at clinicaltrials.gov nets two hundred and twenty-nine studies are completed, underway, or in the works.[139]

Dr. Masino may be the perfect person to write this book. Her position as a professor at a liberal arts college gives her something of a free hand to study a range of interrelated phenomena, seeing the big picture as well as the specific.

***

Clearly, this isn't just some hocus-pocus, read-it-online-somewhere kind of stuff. But there are some very interesting, very passionate people who are moving the work forward. Another speaker at this year's Metabolic Health Summit,

---

138 "Search of: Ketogenic," US National Library of Medicine, National Institutes of Health, PubMed, accessed October 26, 2020.

139 "Search of: Ketogenic," US National Library of Medicine, National Institutes of Health, ClinicalTrials.gov, accessed October 23, 2020.

Mary Newport, MD, had a very personal reason to go down this road.

Dr. Newport's husband Steve was diagnosed Alzheimer's disease at the age of only fifty-four, a grim diagnosis given that Alzheimer's is the most feared disease in America. Diagnoses are rising worldwide at near-epidemic proportions, and there is no known treatment that can cure, or even really treat, the disease.[140]

As Dr. Newport explains, there are several factors influencing the development of Alzheimer's in a patient: age, genetics, and the development of plaque in the brain...these are well-known. What is also well-known, but is only just beginning to be explored, is the connection to metabolism. "There are metabolic factors that we're learning more and more about, insulin resistance being very high on the list. It's been called 'type three diabetes,' or diabetes of the brain."[141]

It's this connection Dr. Newport began to explore when her husband became sicker and sicker. "By the time he was fifty-eight years old, he couldn't use a computer, couldn't do simple math, couldn't read." Desperate to help her husband, Dr. Newport searched for clinical trials and experimental treatments. She read something about a "medical food" being studied for Alzheimer's with some positive results. After a

140 Frederick Kunkle, "Alzheimer's Spurs the Fearful to Change Their Lives to Delay It," *Washington Post*, July 4, 2015.

141 Mary Newport, "Improvement with MCTs and Ketone Monoester in a Case of Alzheimer's: What Happened and Why?" PowerPoint presentation at Metabolic Health Summit, Long Beach CA, January 30–February 2, 2020.

lot of digging, she discovered the food in question was something she was familiar with thanks to her work as a neonatologist: a type of fat called medium-chain triglycerides, or MCTs.

"This was like a perfect storm coming together," she says. "We used to add MCT oil to the feedings of premature babies. Then companies began adding coconut oil and palm kernel oil—which is where MCTs come from—to the formula they produced in order to mimic breast milk, which is very rich in MCT oil." There's good reason for this: "ketones provide 74 percent of the energy to the newborn brain, and they're building blocks for the lipids and cholesterol in the developing brain; so they're very important to the newborn." (In fact, some researchers speculate the reason human infants are born with so much "baby fat," is because those cute little chubs are actually stores of fuel for the child's big ol' brain to develop.)[142]

In her talk, Dr. Newport points to brain scans of people with Alzheimer's showing, as early as their twenties, their brains beginning to lose the ability to use glucose as fuel. However, "the brain has metabolic flexibility" and can continue to use ketones if they are available, even well into the progression of the disease.

She had nothing to lose. She went out and bought some coconut oil and started feeding it to Steve with his breakfast.

---

142 Stephen C. Cunnane and Michael A. Crawford, "Survival of The Fattest: Fat Babies Were the Key to Evolution of the Large Human Brain," *Comparative Biochemistry and Physiology, Part A, Molecular & Integrative Physiology* 136, no. 1 (September 2003): 17-26.

Within days, she documented marked improvements on cognitive screening tests. "Steve said it was like a light bulb came on in his head the day he started coconut oil. He felt that. He went from being very depressed to this mood being elevated and saying he had hope for the future, after just about four or five days."

"From that day on, every morning for breakfast, I gave him that amount. I also started cooking with it—everything was coconut in our house. Flaked coconut, coconut milk...I mean, everything you could think of." She continued to see Steve improve; the life came back into his face, he began whistling again, he regained the ability to read, and could actually remember what he read several hours later.

Ultimately, the disease did take Steve away from her, but she credits her use of MCT oil, and eventually ketone supplements, with giving her a few extra years with her husband. In the twelve years since, Dr. Newport has become a sought-after speaker and has written several books on the metabolic aspects of Alzheimer's. MCT oil and ketones are still not standard treatment for the disease, but she's gratified to see the Alzheimer's Association now recognizes and even funds research studies on the use of ketones.

***

Another passionate scholar of metabolic treatments is Thomas Seyfried, PhD, Professor of Biology at Boston College. His work focuses on the ketogenic diet in the treatment of that emperor of all maladies: cancer. His book *Cancer as a Metabolic Disease* uses case studies in brain cancer patients to argue metabolism is a key to understanding and treating this disease. Again, it's a book written for health professionals and sails way over my head, but lucky for me Dr. Seyfried is an engaging and provocative speaker and interviewee.

Dr. Seyfried sat with Jim Abrahams for a series of short videos for the Charlie Foundation website. He explains that several years ago, he was studying gene expression and cancer in mice at his lab in Boston. One of his students attended a conference on metabolic therapy, "so they came back very enthusiastic about this keto stuff. And I said, well, why not, we had a few extra bucks."[143] They began studying ketosis and seizure control in mice and noticed, regardless of which gene mutation had caused the epilepsy, the ketogenic diet seemed to work.

"It was very funny," he said, "because we were running cancer studies and epilepsy studies simultaneously in the lab—we had a series of brain tumors, and a series of epilepsy mice— and actually the two fields were becoming more and more overlapping in terms of molecular mechanisms." In the cancerous mice, they began to find lowering the amount of glucose in the animal's body would slow the growth of the tumor. "So, we're looking at two phenomena here: the lowering of the glucose and the elevation of the ketones and, in one case, it was managing epileptic seizures; in the other case, it was managing the rate of tumor growth."[144]

---

143 Zupec-Kania, Beth, "Thomas Seyfried, PhD, Professor, Researcher and Pioneer of Cancer as a Metabolic Disease," *Keto Lifestyle* (blog), The Charlie Foundation for Ketogenic Therapies, accessed October 23, 2020.

144 Ibid.

For Dr. Seyfried, a geneticist by training, this was both exciting and challenging. "The NIH says on its website cancer is a genetic disease. If you look at every single textbook—biology, biochemistry—they'll tell you cancer is a genetic disease. The field has been indoctrinated."[145]

But it hadn't always been that way. In 1931, Otto Warburg was awarded the Nobel Prize in physiology or medicine. His work had shown cancerous cells respirate and grow differently than other cells.[146] "Otto Warburg said long ago these tumors are driven by glucose," Dr. Seyfried says, but when American biologist James Watson and English physicist Francis Crick discovered DNA in the 1950s (work for which they were also awarded the Nobel Prize), the entire field of cancer research moved in that direction.[147] Biology "developed a little bit of maturity and sexiness about it, and the field just massively went into looking for gene mutations in cancers, thinking that this was going to be the management of the disease." The hope was, "once we figured out what these mutations did, we'd be able to correct them and correct the cancer."[148]

To this day, Dr. Seyfried says, most of the funding and the research in the field of cancer is going to genetic studies, but these haven't given us much progress in patient outcomes. His experience in his lab made him wonder, "Why isn't it

---

145 Ibid.

146 "Otto Warburg—Facts," Nobel Prize, Nobel Media AB 2020, accessed October 23, 2020.

147 "Francis Crick—Facts," Nobel Prize, Nobel Media AB 2020, accessed October 23, 2020.

148 Zupec-Kania, "Thomas Seyfried, PhD."

more important to figure out how a general therapy might work than trying to pin down genes?"[149]

Since then, he has focused his work on the use of the keto-genic diet in cancer. As he explains, a cancer cell has a muta-tion making it unable to produce energy normally; rather, it has to rely on a process called fermentation. Fermentation involves two fuels: glucose and glutamine. "Both of these fuels impact each other and are powerfully synergistic. When we use keto alone, we shut down the glucose arm of this pathway."[150] This is why the diet can slow, but not completely stop, the growth of a tumor.

Proportion also matters. Some types of cancers are more glucose dependent, while others need more glutamine. Dr. Seyfried gives the example of glioblastoma, a particularly terrible brain cancer: "You have two different kinds of cells: The stem cells, proliferating like crazy, are primarily glucose dependent. But the highly invasive mesenchymal neoplastic cells are more glutamine dependent than glucose dependent." In the "press-pulse" strategy he and his team have pioneered, "What we do is simply target both, and we'll kill both cell types."[151]

The treatment is not being used widely, but he believes it holds promise.[152] As he and his co-authors ask in the title of

---

149 Ibid.

150 Ibid.

151 Ibid.

152 Thomas N, Seyfried et al, "Press-Pulse: A Novel Therapeutic Strategy for the Metabolic Management of Cancer," *Nutrition & metabolism* 14 no. 19. (February 23, 2017)

a recent in the journal *Neurochemical Research*, "Provocative Question: Should Ketogenic Metabolic Therapy Become the Standard of Care for Glioblastoma?"[153]

The current standard of care—usually involving some combination of chemo and radiation—is wrongheaded, Dr. Seyfried believes. "You're treating people based on therapies that are not related to the origin or the management of the disease. You can kill cancer cells by poisoning somebody. I mean, you can incinerate their whole organ with radiation. But these poor people are put at massive risk for other kinds of things down the road. Why would you want to do that if you could achieve the same end goal with another approach?"

Again, diet therapy is not currently a standard treatment. Vinnie Tortorich's story aside, few doctors would use it in their practice or recommend it to their patients. Still, other researchers are exploring the ketogenic diet as an adjuvant, or additional therapy, to help make the standard treatments more effective. More news about this may be coming soon.

***

Not to be outdone, our four-legged friends are getting in on the act. I had the opportunity to consider Dr. Seyfried's ideas last year when my ten-year-old dog Jake was diagnosed with adenocarcinoma, a form of cancer in the anal gland. I remember when we got the diagnosis. I spent countless late-night hours on sites like PetMD reading things like, "While

---

153 Thomas N. Seyfried et al, "Provocative Question: Should Ketogenic Metabolic Therapy Become the Standard of Care for Glioblastoma?" *Neurochemical Research* 44 (October 2019): 2392–2404.

anal gland/sac cancer is not common; it is an invasive disease that does not generally have a positive outlook," and "Due to the type of disease, it is typically malignant and can spread quickly into other areas of the animal's body."[154] It was scary stuff.

Judy and I make no bones about the fact we baby our pup, and we were committed to doing all we could to help him. We found the best veterinary oncologist in the area (yep, that's a thing), and booked surgery and chemo as soon as possible. During our consultation, I asked the vet about what to be feeding our little guy. Sure enough, she advised we find a dog food with a low carbohydrate content, and she recommended a couple of brands.

After surgery, a course of chemo, and now maintenance medication, Jake is doing well—still taking hikes, still playing, still loving life the way only a crazy Jack Russell can. At every check-up, the doctor is impressed by how well he's doing and how so far we've been able to manage the disease.

Our vet is not the only one who's onto this secret. The KetoPet Sanctuary is a nonprofit founded in 2014 with the mission "to give shelter dogs with terminal cancer a 'forever home' and save them from euthanization." Some of the dogs brought to the fifty-three-acre Texas ranch have been given only a week to live, but all are given the best care available, along with a ketogenic diet.[155]

---

154 "Anal Gland Cancer in Dogs," PetMD, July 2, 2008.

155 "Our Beginning: A Keto Sanctuary for Dogs with Cancer," KetoPet: About Us, accessed October 23, 2020.

The outcomes are remarkable. According to their website, "55 percent of the dogs who graduated from the KPS program are still going for long walks, enjoying belly rubs, eating a raw keto diet, and experiencing a quality of life far beyond their original prognosis."[156] In a 2019 article published in the journal *Innovative Veterinary Care*, the KetoPet team presented a series of case studies representing some of the dramatic results in their patients. The article concludes, "The KetoPet team of veterinary oncologists and research scientists gained unprecedented insights from addressing cancer as a disease of metabolism. Incorporating this approach with standard of care offers a new potential for dogs to live long vibrant lives."[157]

***

I was able to catch up with Dr. Rho, whose talk I quoted at the start of this chapter. Dr. Rho's publications include textbooks on both epilepsy medications and the many forms of dietary therapy. He emphasizes although diet is not the one and only answer (after all, there are still many patients for whom diet doesn't work), we need to acknowledge the historical bias against diet as a medical treatment. "For decades, the paradigm for drug discovery in Western medicine has been understanding the science and biology in order to find a therapeutic target—what they call a 'druggable' target." However, in epilepsy, Alzheimer's, and other conditions, this approach hasn't yielded much progress. "There are many more drugs

---

156 Ibid.

157 Chelsea Kent et al, "KetoPet Sanctuary: Ketosis, Cancer and Canines—Part 2," *Innovative Veterinary Care*, June 25, 2019.

now than there were one-hundred years ago, but the overall efficacy rates haven't changed. We still have about a third of epilepsy patients that don't respond to any drugs at all."

In a larger sense, Dr. Rho believes dietary intervention may represent "a paradigm shift, in terms of how we do drug discovery." He says although there's a lot more work to be done, "the ketogenic diet—and metabolic therapy as a whole—has implications and ramifications for general health. We're in a very different climate today, and in the next hundred years of dietary therapy we should think more broadly about the potential benefits and evaluate them objectively, free from historical bias" to continue to move medical research forward.

***

The ketogenic diet might not be a magic diet, but it sure seems to have a lot of potential, particularly for those who want to be free from disease. That's not to say it is for everyone. I have friends who do very well on other diets: vegetarian, pescatarian, flexitarian, carno-, ovo-, lacto-, pesco-, pollo-tarians, and so on. One thing most all of these folks agree on, though, is food matters. You don't have to go it alone; as we've seen, finding a tribe or a team is an important aspect of finding your own path to health. There's one person, though, you should always have on your team: a good primary care doctor.

CHAPTER 17

PRIMARY CARE: THE POWER OF PARTNERSHIP

———

Where do you go when you're sick? That's easy: the doctor. But where do you go when healthcare itself is sick? That one is much tougher.

Here in the US, we have an interesting phrase in our healthcare system: primary care. According to the American Academy of Family Physicians, "A primary care physician is a specialist in family medicine, internal medicine, or pediatrics who provides definitive care to the undifferentiated patient at the point of first contact and *takes continuing responsibility for providing the patient's comprehensive care*" (emphasis mine).[158]

———

158 "All Policies: Primary Care," American Association of Family Physicians, accessed October 23, 2020.

But let's think about this a minute. When I'm teaching my students in a freshman English class, I help them understand the definition of what is called primary research—research you conduct yourself. Interviewing people, writing and distributing a survey, making observations, doing experiments in a lab...all of these, I tell them, are examples of primary research.

Secondary research—which freshmen writers spend a lot more time doing—is reading and listening to what others say, like one would find in articles, case studies, white papers... it's when you turn to the experts, find out what they have to say, and use their ideas to help to solve a problem.

Too often, it seems, "primary care" is when we go to the doctor and ask them to use their expertise to make a pronouncement on what's going on with our bodies and brains. We ask for their solutions to the problem in the form of a drug, procedure, or device. But doesn't this sound more like the *secondary* research my students are doing?

What if we take back this phrase, "primary care?" What if "primary care" is the care we give ourselves? The levers we pull to make ourselves feel good, perform well, and live happy, healthy lives? What if, instead of the physician "taking continuing responsibility" for our health, we all step up and take ownership of that responsibility?

It's a small change, but one opening up many possibilities. We have one body, one brain, and one life. It's ours to keep— to have and to hold, in sickness and health, for better or worse, 'til death do we part, just like a loved one or a child.

And yet, many of us who take these other responsibilities with the utmost care and seriousness treat this care of our primary selves as secondary, even frivolous.

∗∗∗

But maybe there's a third way. Maybe the best results come when the primary care*giver* joins forces with the primary care physician, drawing on that doctor's expertise but still taking responsibility for making the changes needed to optimize our health. This is what the AAFP calls "the role of patient as partner in health care."[159] The model of care used by epilepsy diet centers like Dr. Hughes's and Dr. Cervenka's points to some interesting possibilities, such as breaking down barriers between specialists and using different forms of expertise and outreach to extend medicine into their patients' lives. But a few doctors are taking this idea one step further.

Brian Lenzkes, MD, is one of the voices of the *Low Carb MD Podcast* and one of the doctors looking at our healthcare system with a 30,000-foot view to find ways to fix it. He and his cohost Dr. Tro Kalaysian have each created their practices around a new model called direct primary care.

Dr. Lenzkes was kind enough to speak with me early on a Tuesday morning. The difference between the side-by-side screens on my computer couldn't be more pronounced. Here on the East Coast, it was nine o'clock on a cool, gray morning, my sluggish mood even further dampened by the

---

159 Ibid.

recent discovery I'd run out of coffee. Meanwhile Dr. Lenz-kes, calling in from San Diego—where it was *six o'clock in the morning*, mind you—was all smiles, laughing good-naturedly, and talking rapidly and energetically. He seemed for all the world like a kid on Christmas morning.

Even more interesting, though, is the contrast to the last time I saw Dr. Lenzkes on screen at this year's Low Carb USA virtual conference back in the summer. At the time, his demeanor was grave, and his voice was deep and gravelly, as befitting of his topic: physician burnout.[160]

"There's a silent epidemic in healthcare," his talk began. After briefly defining burnout ("long-term, unresolved, job-related stress that leads to exhaustion, cynicism, feelings of detachment from one's job responsibilities, and lack of a sense of persona accomplishment"), Dr. Lenzkes shared some startling statistics:[161]

- National studies suggest 50 percent of doctors in the US meet the criteria for burnout.
- According to the Medscape National Physician Burnout and Suicide Report 2020, up to 77 percent of doctors reported their work had a negative impact on their relationships.
- The average internal medicine doctor takes care of 2500 patients. To provide the recommended level of care to

---

160 Brian Lenzkes, "Physician Burnout: The Silent Epidemic in Healthcare," PowerPoint presentation at Low Carb USA Virtual San Diego 2020 Conference, August 27, 2020.

161 Ibid.

that many patients, that doctor would need to work 21.7 hours per day.

- The suicide rate among male doctors is 40 percent higher than it is for the general population. Among female doctors, it's 130 percent higher.
- On average, 300 physicians commit suicide each year. If each of these is seeing 2000 patients, then this means 600,000 people each year are affected by physician suicide.
- Still, these doctors are less likely to seek psychological help than most people.

In his talk, Dr. Lenzkes spoke frankly about his own experience as a physician of seventeen years: "It feels like you're on a treadmill that's moving way too fast." Each year, he said, there seemed to be more bureaucracy, more paperwork, and less autonomy. It's a confluence of factors: ever-shrinking reimbursements from insurance companies and from Medicare and Medicaid means doctors need to see more patients just to make ends meet, patients losing insurance and becoming sicker every year, and stringent documentation requirements meaning more and more forms for doctors to fill out.

"I have always loved patient interactions," he tells me, "but I hated having to do prior authorizations all day long, trying to beg the insurance company for a medicine that was needed or a sleep study, or a colonoscopy, or whatever it was." All of the paperwork and all of the begging would cut into the time he could spend with patients. "If you ask many doctors, they'll tell you they can only spend about six to eight minutes per patient."

The treadmill was going faster and faster, and Dr. Lenzkes began to worry he would never catch up: "I didn't want to be someone who's just working for a paycheck, but I graduated from medical school with $300,000 in student loans. Here I am, fifty years old, and I still haven't paid them off."

***

On top of these struggles, Dr. Lenzkes had his own health problems. "Two years ago, I was forty pounds heavier than I am now. Here I am, eating six small meals throughout the day, I'm exercising six days a week and each year I'm gaining three, five, seven, ten pounds."[162]

One day, a patient came in having lost a significant amount of weight on his own. The patient told him he had read Dr. Fung's book, so Dr. Lenzkes looked into it. "I started realizing...gosh I've been giving bad advice, and I've been given bad advice. I said if this guy Fung is right, I'm going to be super mad because everything I've been doing has been detrimental."

But sure enough, when he tried restricting his carbs, it worked. "Dr. Fung says you can't throw drugs at a lifestyle problem. It makes so much sense." His patients, noticing his weight loss, began to ask about his secret. More and more often, he found himself teaching them about lifestyle, rather than simply prescribing drugs. Dr. Lenzkes points out the word "doctor" comes from the Latin "docere" meaning "to teach," and he

---

162 Bret Scher, "Diet Doctor Podcast #41—Brian Lenzkes," March 11, 2020, on *Diet Doctor Podcast*, podcast, MP3 audio, 54:25.

found it satisfying to be able to teach his patients to heal themselves through lifestyle and so gratifying when patients were able reverse their diabetes and other health conditions through diet. "I found myself actually taking patients *off* medications. I'd never seen that before."

It came at a cost, though. Spending more time with his patients meant, "I had to bust my butt, work through lunch every day, and work late trying to help people." Every day would stretch to fourteen hours—with a forty-minute commute besides. "My neighbors were teasing me, saying, 'You don't have to wash your car because we never see it. It's dark when you leave and dark when you come home.'" Weekends were spent catching up on notes from the week and preparing for the following week.

Nor did it always work. "My reality—a lot of doctors' reality—is 80 percent of people don't really care about their health, 20 percent you can really invest in and help, and so eighty percent of the time you're really wasting your time trying to teach them."

***

One day flying home from a conference, he had a realization. There were two flight attendants on the plane. One was kind, smiling, and chatting with the passengers, while the other seemed just to be going through the motions. "I said, man, she must hate her job. She's here for the same amount of time, but maybe she's just burned out." When the attendant read the safety announcement, Dr. Lenzkes looked around and noticed no one was listening to her. "I said, you know what, she's kind of like me. I'm trying to tell people, 'Hey, you're at risk of diabetes.' But they don't really care, until it actually happens. Then they want me to fix the problem right away."

"Then she said to put your own oxygen mask on, and I said, 'You know what, I'm not putting my own oxygen mask on. I'm watching my diet, I'm exercising, sure. But I'm stressed, running around, not getting sleep...I know all these things can affect metabolic health, so why am I doing it?'"

Later that day, the comparison became even clearer. "The pilot is standing there while I'm leaving the plane, and I'm not even paying attention. Why? Because I'm on the phone, trying to get my stuff, get my life arranged, and get off the plane; I've got a lot to do...and I realize I walked right by the pilot. Here's this guy who risked his life to get me to my destination on time; he was away from his family and his kids... and I realized I never even said thank you. I thought, 'how many people say thank you to me?' It's not as common as you might think. Especially in those types of practices where the doctor has to rush people through and can't establish a relationship with the patient."

He was tired of the proverbial treadmill. His cohost Dr. Tro talked him into trying a new kind of approach. "He goes, 'Brian, what are you doing, man? You're killing yourself and you're not as effective as you can be." Dr.Lenzkes was ready to listen. "I just realized the futility of my situation. I was tired of being a workhorse."

The model Dr. Tro had established at his own practice in New York, and which Dr. Lenzkes began to look into, was direct primary care. Rather than the traditional model in which a doctor is paid per-visit using a pre-negotiated rate with an insurance company, direct primary care is more of a subscription model, in which patients pay a monthly fee (in Dr. Lenzkes's practice, one hundred to one hundred and fifty dollars per month) that covers as many visits as they need, plus any necessary tests, equipment, and so on. He describes it as being similar to AAA, the auto club. "You always hope you don't need it, but when you do need it, it's there for you right away."

He began the Low Carb MD San Diego practice in July, with a special focus on metabolic health. Dr. Lenzkes admits although his income may not be what it was, his quality of life has improved vastly. His patient load has gone from two thousand to just two hundred and fifty. He works regular hours, has an office just minutes from his home, and gets to spend time with his family again. "Now I have to wash my car," he laughs. "My neighbors say, 'Oh you actually live there, huh?'"

But the direct primary care model is even more beneficial for those two hundred and fifty patients. They don't have to wait months just to get an appointment. When they do see him, they get to spend more time with Dr. Lenzkes in each visit. This enables him to talk to his patients, listen to them, and teach them. He's also able to order tests an insurance company might not cover, like insulin levels, and in doing so, provide much more individualized care for each patient. "I can take a group of patients out for a walk at lunch time. We spend an hour talking about their lives, their struggles, and in addition to just getting to know them and establishing that relationship, I can help them think of ways to improve their lifestyle."

Dr. Lenzkes brought on board a partner, Dr. Kristen Baier, who used a ketogenic diet to manage her own health issues such as migraines, lupus, and autoimmune disease. She was eager to join his practice, she says, because in her previous life working for a medical device company, "I really for the first time saw the business side of medicine and how it does not focus on the wellbeing of the patient. A lot of it is financially driven." She says although there are a lot of good doctors doing good work for their patients, there are pressures and incentives within the system helping to drive up the high cost of health care. "It was really eye-opening." At this new practice, she says, "I want to bring integrity back to medicine."

In an interview with Dr. Tro Kalayjian on the *Low Carb MD Podcast,* Dr. Baier gave a startling glimpse into the life of a doctor in a hospital system. "When we worked in urgent care, some days we had over eighty patients; we'd be expected to see over eighty patients in a twelve-hour shift. It gets unsafe. You can't provide quality care when you only have ten minutes with a patient, and then you're spending two hours every evening catching up on labs and returning calls. It's just a horrible system. Patients are not happy. Doctors are not happy. In the meantime, the health care administration is getting million-dollar bonuses every year on the back of the work you're doing. It has to change."[163]

---

163 Brian Lenzkes and Tro Kalayjian, MD, "Episode 109: Dr. Kristin Baier," May 27, 2020, in *Low Carb MD Podcast*, podcast, MP3 audio, 47:02.

Nor is there much freedom or autonomy for doctors these days, even if they had the ability to do so. Dr. Baier said, "Patients don't realize that if we don't follow the templates that support the pharmaceutical companies, we get penalized." I am reminded once again of Jim Abrahams's bold statement that "there are powerful forces in the healthcare system that have nothing to do with health."

Dr. Baier was thrilled to join Dr. Lenzkes in the new venture. The growing Low Carb MD team now includes a health coach, a physical trainer, a nutritionist, and more. According to Dr. Lenzkes, "The most frustrating thing for a patient is when you tell them to lower their carbs, but then they go see a nutritionist and the nutritionist says, 'No, that doctor is crazy.' When we get everybody on the same page, it makes such a difference for the patient."

***

The other thing Dr. Lenzkes and Dr. Baier are able to do is to leverage the power of technology. "We can give our patients a bluetooth scale, a smart blood pressure cuff, and a continuous glucose monitor," Dr. Lenzkes says. A continuous glucose monitor, or CGM, is a small wearable device which tracks a person's blood sugar levels throughout the day. "These report right back to my phone, so if I see someone's blood sugar out of control, I can reach out to them and say 'Hey, what's going on?' Maybe they indulged in a piece of cake, or maybe they're going through a lot of stress or sleeplessness. I can help the patient right away, instead of waiting three months until I get to see them again."

It's a new kind of house call, if you will, and a way of closing the loop of lifestyle medicine. Perhaps for people with epilepsy, it might move the needle on that 50 percent compliance rate.[164]

I'm reminded of an old quote by motivational speaker Zig Ziglar: "People often say that motivation doesn't last. Well, neither does bathing—that's why we recommend it daily."[165] Nowhere is this truer than in lifestyle changes like diet and exercise. In my own experience, I do pretty well at staying the course, but my eating two days before and after my appointment with Dr. Cervenka and Bobbie is the cleanest I ever do. I have to think the kinds of interventions that Dr. Lenzkes and Dr. Baier are using—from their team to their tech—would help me to keep on point, week after week.

But Dr. Lenzkes, Dr. Baier, and Dr. Kalayjian are in San Diego, Chicago, and New York, respectively. What to do? I've done my best to recreate that model. Using the directory on the Low Carb USA website, I found a primary care doctor who understands and supports this diet. She's a smart, thoughtful, caring physician who believes in always learning and who works hard to provide an excellent level of care within the confines of the conventional system. Every time she runs tests, I ask her to forward the results to Dr. Cervenka to keep everyone on the same "team." I've found coaching support through an app, which includes diet and exercise tracking tools, plus regular text check-ins and phone calls

164 Fang Ye et al, "Efficacy of and Patient Compliance with a Ketogenic Diet in Adults with Intractable Epilepsy: A Meta-Analysis," *Journal of Clinical Neurology* 11 no. 1 (January 2015): 26-31.

165 "Zig Ziglar Quotes," BrainyQuote, accessed October 23, 2020.

with a coach. I've also joined Dr. Tro Kalayjian's weekly Zoom town hall sessions.

"These meetings were organized shortly after the COVID-19 pandemic struck, and we became aware of the additional stresses and challenges faced by patients trying to maintain their low-carb lifestyle." Dr. Tro writes.[166] In his practice, he saw a big surge in patients asking for anxiety medications, gaining weight, or resorting to old patterns. "We knew we had to do something," he says. The sessions have morphed into a group coaching program: a weekly virtual support group in which Dr. Tro and his two health coaches share research along with practical tips for staying the course in challenging times. Participants share their own experiences and ask questions of the experts. It's an incredibly supportive atmosphere, and I always walk away inspired and comforted.

***

So why isn't this the norm? According to Dr. Lenzkes, there's a structural problem when insurance companies hold the reins and doctors are paid per visit, per procedure, or per test. Under the old model, "unfortunately, the sicker the patient got, the more money I'd make," Dr. Lenzkes says. "If a patient uses lifestyle to improve their health, I lose out."

"Insurance companies don't see the time we invest in education as being valuable," he laments, so instead of addressing

---

166 Chris S. Cornell, "Online Group Coaching Aims to Help Participants Maintain Benefits of Low Carb & Fasting; Manage Stress During These Difficult Times," Doctor Tro's Medical Weight Loss and Direct Primary Care, April 30, 2020.

problems early, "we wait until you blow up your engine. Then we say, 'Well yeah, you blew up your engine, so now we have to do a bypass surgery.' What could we have done to prevent that ten years ago?"

Perhaps the problem is one of perspective. It seems to me our medical care system was built for acute, not chronic diseases. If you have a sore throat, a six-to-eight-minute consult may be all you need to find out whether it's strep. If you fall and hurt your foot, a doctor can diagnose within six to eight minutes whether it's broken or merely sprained. But chronic diseases—lifestyle diseases like obesity, diabetes, heart disease—take years to develop and years to correct. Our healthcare system just isn't built to handle that. Meanwhile, chronic disease rates continue to rise, and costs spiral out of control. A recent review estimates chronic disease drives approximately 75 percent of healthcare costs in the United States.[167]

The world of medicine hasn't evolved to catch up with this epidemic. As Dr. Lenzkes says, we don't have a good prevention system in place, so when problems appear, we wait until they develop into acute problems, which are more expensive to treat. All those engines blowing out, when all we really needed to do was to replace a few gaskets early on. Going back to his AAA analogy, Dr. Lenzkes says, "It only works if everyone keeps their car in shape. If everyone's car breaks down every day, then the company goes out of business. In medicine that's happening now. Everyone's getting sicker

167 Timothy B. Norbeck, "Drivers of Health Care Costs. A Physicians Foundation White Paper—Second of a Three-Part Series," *Missouri Medicine* 110, no. 2 (March–April 2013): 113-8.

and sicker. Why? We're not addressing the root cause of all these problems, which is metabolic disease."[168]

***

What's the solution? How can a model like direct primary care become the norm rather than the exception? Dr. Lenzkes says the best hope may be not in convincing health insurance companies but in convincing their counterparts. "Guess who's going to be more interested in this stuff than anyone? It's not the health insurance companies, it's the life insurance companies because they're interested in clients living longer. In our practice, we're looking at longevity and trying to help people live the best lives they can. The more active they are, the less stressed they are, the more they're sleeping...all those ways we can intervene are going to make a long-term, tangible difference when the patients are eighty years old and they're still playing tennis. I mean, that's a person who's not going to be in the hospital every week. Really, we're looking at, how we can help you age the best you can."

It's a crazy idea, paying doctors to keep people healthy rather than merely to treat sickness. But it's the change we need in order to address the massive health problems we're seeing today—and the resultant financial problems.

Ben Bocchiccio, PhD, fitness and exercise expert shared a powerful graphic during his talk at this year's Low Carb USA virtual conference. It's a picture of a half-circle fuel gauge

168 Brian Sanders and Brian Lenzkes, "The Future of Medicine, Aligning Incentives, and Fixing the Broken Healthcare (Sickcare) System," June 23, 2020, in *Peak Human*, podcast, MP3 audio, 1:20:14.

like you'd see in your car, with the title "Illness to Health Continuum." Next to the left side of the scale, "E" is replaced with the word "Illness." Instead of "F" on the right is the word "Health." At the top of the arc—somewhere in between illness and health—is the phrase, "Absence of Disease."[169]

"Most doctors deal with illness," Dr. Bocchicchio says, "and their goal is to get their patients to an absence-of-disease state...even though absence of disease may be, in modern-day medicine, someone who's taking two or three prescription drugs." He wants more for his clients to get them all the way to full health. "Health is vibrance. Health is vitality. Health is a high level of functioning."[170]

For Dr. Bocchicchio, the key to health is metabolism, and the key to metabolism is lifestyle. Outsiders like Dr. Lenzkes, Dr. Baier, and Dr. Kalayjian are innovating to find new ways to help their patients enact lifestyle change. In their practices, in their practices, in their podcast, and on social media, they are building communities and supporting others—both their patients and their listeners—in each individual's journey to change their mindset, sustain their motivation, and find empowerment through the journey toward health.

"Let food be thy medicine," is a quote often attributed to Hippocrates. It could be food—along with stress, sleep, exercise, community, and mindset—is not just the past, but the future of medicine as well. But practices like Dr. Lenzkes's can't

---

169 Ben Bocchicchio, "The Power of The Muscle System in The Management of Metabolic Dysfunction," PowerPoint presentation at Low Carb USA Virtual San Diego 2020 Conference, August 28, 2020.

170 Ibid.

become the norm if only twenty percent of us are willing to step up and accept that challenge. We all need to embrace lifestyle and ask our practitioners to do the same in order for the system to change. The health of healthcare, and along with it the health of our economy and the health of our country as a whole, depends on it. If we do, we may learn just how powerful we are.

AFTERWORD:
A PUBLIC SERVICE
ANNOUNCEMENT

———

Ken Jeong is an American actor, comedian, and very funny person. He's famous for the TV series *Community* and movies like *The Hangover* and *Crazy Rich Asians*. He's also a medical doctor.

So, I was a little surprised during his recent stand-up special *You Complete Me, Ho*, when he told the story of an audience member having a severe, generalized tonic-clonic seizure at one of his shows. He described going right back into doctor mode, running toward the patient to help. But the hero of the story is fellow comedian Ice Cube, whom Jeong calls "the baddest motherfucker on the planet." Ice Cube also rushed toward the scene, Jeong said, and "we're like two outfielders running for the same ball."[171]

———

171 Ken Jeong, *You Complete Me, Ho*, Netflix Special, 2019.

Seeing that Ice Cube is taking off his belt, "I'm like, 'Whoa! You don't whip the patient, Cube!'" But Ice Cube arrives before Jeong does and puts the belt into the patient's mouth, so the person "doesn't choke on his tongue."

In the special, the audience erupts into applause as Jeong concludes, "Ice Cube, not me, saved the patient's life."

Okay, now I know Jeong's standup doesn't constitute medical advice—it's hard to imagine anything further from it—and in fact, part of Jeong's act is about how he wasn't a very *good* doctor. Also, the last thing I want to do is hate on the very funny Ken Jeong or the quick-thinking Ice Cube (who indeed is still "the baddest motherfucker on the planet"). But when I saw that special the other night, I felt I had to add one more thing to this book.

So, here's my public service announcement: given one in ten of us will have a seizure at some point in our lifetimes, the chances are pretty good you'll at least witness a grand mal someday. When you do, here's what to do, according to the CDC:[172]

- Ease the person to the floor.
- Turn the person gently onto one side. This will help the person breathe.
- Clear the area around the person of anything hard or sharp. This can prevent injury.

---

172 "Seizure First Aid," Centers for Disease Control and Prevention, last modified September 30, 2020.

- Put something soft and flat, like a folded jacket, under his or her head.
- Remove eyeglasses.
- Loosen ties or anything around the neck that may make it hard to breathe.
- Time the seizure. Call 911 if the seizure lasts longer than five minutes, in the case of repeated seizures or if the person has never had a seizure before.

Here's what NOT to do:

- Do **not** hold the person down or try to stop his or her movements.
- Do **not** put anything in the person's mouth. This can injure teeth or the jaw. A person having a seizure cannot swallow his or her tongue.
- Do **not** try to give mouth-to-mouth breaths (like CPR). People usually start breathing again on their own after a seizure.
- Do **not** offer the person water or food until he or she is fully alert.

Okay, that's my PSA for the day. Thanks for listening.

Be well and live large,

Big Dave

ACKNOWLEDGMENTS

When I first started this crazy project, my professor and mentor Eric Koester said, contrary to popular belief, a book is a collaborative effort, not a solo venture. I had no idea how right he was. So many people made this book possible, and I'm extraordinarily grateful to them all. In particular, I'd like to express my gratitude to all the people who have inspired, motivated, and helped me along the way:

To my reader community, for keeping me accountable and giving me invaluable material and moral support in this journey: my mom and number-one "superfan," Jane Moore Robinson; my dad and "old pal" John B. Robinson, Jr.; my forever-young uncle Carl "Chad" Chadburn; my dear friend, teammate, and fellow book lover Ed Salt; the amazing Jim Abrahams, whose words and generosity inspired this crazy little book; my second family, Benjamin and Nelia Geli, Effie and Romer Geocadin (without whom this book would be very short, indeed), Alvin and Rita Geli, Troy and Pawee Lainson, and Dino and Cathy Geli; my good buddy Bing Cheng; reigning Couple of the Year Jim and Mary Swartz; my dear friends and amazing rescue squad Bill and Jane

Yeingst and Richard LaFace and Patricia Harris; Richard LaFace again, because he's that big of a deal; the indefatigable Cindy and James Caple; fellow upstaters JJ and Pat Miller; my oldest friend and longtime co-conspirator Brian Giering; Guia Llamas; my friend, colleague and car ride confidant Michael Suwak; cousin Catherine Moore; cousins Timothy and Tressa Bruess; nieces and Instagram celebrities Camille Sanchez and Karmina Sanchez; Robin Resteghini; Pamela Zitron; Dino "Cus" Cusumano; my sister, producer, and accountability partners Leanne and Justin Maine; poet-hero Marty Moran; teammate Joe Green; Michele Mintling; my dear sistah and brother Claire and Todd Powers; mentor Eric Koester; practically-niece Anela Sarabia; cousin Minott Osborn; coach and gentleman-scholar Alan Weatherley; Mayra Perez; Daniel Martin; the amazing Jade Nelson; Lala Balaoghlanova; and the incomparable Molly Reid. The world is one small book richer because of all of you.

To my family, who have shaped me into who I am today: my siblings John Paul, Claire, Leanne, Greg, and Peter, whose mixture of love, support, and good-natured ribbing taught me to roll with whatever life threw my way; my aunts and uncles and cousins, who taught how full of humor and joy life can be; my father, who taught me the power of a good one-liner and the pride of a job well done; and most of all (as promised since I was ten years old)..."Thanks, Mom, for putting up with my corny jokes for all those years!"

To my writing teachers: Ruth Vinz, Steven Schwartz, Judy Doenges Leslee Becker, Gerald Callahan and David Mogen, and my longtime mentor and advocate David Milofsky.

To the wonderful folks I've worked with at Georgetown and at New Degree Press, especially Brian Bies, who took a chance on me; David Grandouiller, who helped me iron out the ideas; and Christy Mossburg, who dragged me kicking and screaming across the finish line.

Finally—always and forever—to Judy, my muse, my cheerleader, my fellow misadventurer, my heart. A year ago you said to me, "Hey, there's this professor at Georgetown who runs a book-writing class." Without you, this book would not exist. You are the real hero of this story.

APPENDIX

———

INTRODUCTION

Centers for Disease Control and Prevention. "Chronic Diseases in America." Last modified September 24, 2020. *https://www.cdc. gov/chronicdisease/resources/infographic/chronic-diseases.htm*

CHAPTER 1

Brown, Daniel James. *The Boys in the Boat: Nine Americans and their Epic Quest for Gold at the 1936 Berlin Olympics."* New York: Viking, 2013.

"Exercising and Socializing Can Lead to Better Mental Health." November 7, 2013, in *Health in a Heartbeat.* Produced by UF Health Podcasts. Podcast. MP3 audio. *https://podcasts.ufhealth. org/exercising-and-socializing-can-lead-to-better-mental-health/*

McGonigal, Kelly, Ph.D. *The Joy of Movement.* New York: Penguin Random House, 2019. Kindle.

Rodio, Michael. "Washington, DC Is America's Fittest City for 2016." *Men's Journal,* Accessed October 22, 2020. *https://www.*

mensjournal.com/health-fitness/washington-dc-americas-fit-test-city-2016/

CHAPTER 2

Mann, Traci. "Oprah's Investment in Weight Watchers Was Smart Because the Program Doesn't Work." *Brow Beat* (blog). *Slate*, November 3, 2015 *https://slate.com/culture/2015/11/why-weight-watchers-doesn-t-work.html*

Tortorich, Vinnie with Andy Schreiber. "Throwback: On the Road, Young and Obese." October 12, 2015. in *Fitness Confidential Podcast*. Produced by Vinnie Tortorich. Podcast, MP3 Audio, 6:01. *https://vinnietortorich.com/2019/04/throwback-young-obese-stolen-good-intentions-episode-1300/*

Tortorich, Vinnie with Anna Vocino. "Listener Questions." February 9, 2015. in *Fitness Confidential Podcast*. Produced by Vinnie Tortorich. Podcast, MP3 Audio, 8:45. *https://vinnietortorich.com/2015/02/angriest-trainer-344-listener-questions/*

Tortorich, Vinnie with Dean Lorey. *Fitness Confidential*. Read by the author. Los Angeles: Pistachio Press, 2013. Audible audio ed., 7hr., 16min.

USDA Economic Research Service. "Organic Market Overview." Organic Agriculture. Last modified September 10, 2020. *https://www.ers.usda.gov/topics/natural-resources-environment/organic-agriculture/organic-market-overview.aspx*

CHAPTER 3

Banting, William. "Letter on Corpulence, Addressed to the Public." Internet Archive. London: Harrison, January 1, 1864. Accessed October 22, 2020. *https://archive.org/details/letteroncorpulenoobant/page/8/mode/2up?q=claret.*

Perry, Susan. "Carbs, not fats (nor gluttony, nor sloth) are what's making us fat, says author of controversial new book." *MinnPost*, January 26, 2011. *https://www.minnpost.com/second-opinion/2011/01/carbs-not-fats-nor-gluttony-nor-sloth-are-whats-making-us-fat-says-author-con/*

Taubes, Gary. "Obesity's 'No There There' Problem: A History of Causal Thinking in the Science." Presented at the Low Carb USA Virtual San Diego 2020 Conference, August 29, 2020. *https://www.lowcarbusa.org/videos/premium-event-videos/virtual-san-diego-2020-livestream/*

Taubes, Gary. *Why We Get Fat: And What to Do About It.* (New York: Alfred A. Knopf, 2011).

CHAPTER 4

"6 Years After *The Biggest Loser*, Metabolism Is Slower and Weight Is Back Up." *Scientific American*. May 11, 2016. *https://www.scientificamerican.com/article/6-years-after-the-biggest-loser-metabolism-is-slower-and-weight-is-back-up/*

Beck, Leslie. "I Have Low Blood Sugar—What Should I Eat?" *The Globe and Mail*, May 30, 2012. *https://www.theglobeandmail.com/life/health-and-fitness/ask-a-health-expert/i-have-low-blood-sugar---what-should-i-eat/article4217681/*

Centers for Disease Control and Prevention. "Obesity and Overweight." FastStats—Overweight Prevalence, Last modified February 28, 2020 *https://www.cdc.gov/nchs/fastats/obesity-overweight.htm*

Fung, Jason, M.D. "My Single Best Weight-Loss Tip." Diet Doctor. November 4, 2018. Accessed October 22, 2020. *https://www.dietdoctor.com/my-single-best-weight-loss-tip*

Fung, Jason, M.D. *The Obesity Code: Unlocking the Secrets of Weight Loss*. Read by Brian Nishii. New York: Greystone Books, 2016. Audible audio ed. 10 hrs., 9 min.

Kalayjian, Tro, MD and Brian Lenzkes, MD. "Episode 110: Dr. Ben Bikman is Back!" June 1, 2020. In *Low Carb MD Podcast*. Podcast, MP3 audio. *https://lowcarbmd.com/episode-110-dr-ben-bikman-is-back*

Last, Allen R., M.D., M.P.H., and Stephen A. Wilson, M.D., M.P.H. "Low-Carbohydrate Diets." *American Family Physician* 73, no. 11 (June 2006); 1942-1948 *https://www.aafp.org/afp/2006/0601/p1942.html*

McDonalds. "Nutrition Calculator." last accessed October 22, 2020. *https://www.mcdonalds.com/us/en-us/about-our-food/nutrition-calculator.html*

Melzer, Katarina. "Carbohydrate and Fat Utilization During Rest and Physical Activity." *Clinical Nutrion Espen* 6 no. 2 (Apri 2011): E45-E52. *https://doi.org/10.1016/j.eclnm.2011.01.005*

Nikols-Richardson, Sharon M, PhD, RD, Mary Dean Coleman, PhD, RD, Joanne J. Volpe, and Kathy W. Hosig, PhD, MPH, RD. "Perceived Hunger Is Lower and Weight Loss Is Greater in Overweight Premenopausal Women Consuming a Low-Carbohydrate/High-Protein vs High-Carbohydrate/Low-Fat Diet." *Journal of the American Dietetic Association* 105 no. 9 (September 2005): 1433-1437 *https://doi.org/10.1016/j.jada.2005.06.025*

Office of Disease Prevention and Health Promotion. "Appendix 7. Nutritional Goals for Age-Sex Groups Based on Dietary Reference Intakes and Dietary Guidelines Recommendations," Dietary Guidelines 2015-2020. Accessed October 22, 2020 *https://health.gov/our-work/food-nutrition/2015-2020-dietary-guidelines/guidelines/appendix-7/*

Taubes, Gary. *Why We Get Fat: And What to Do About It.* (New York: Alfred A. Knopf, 2011).

Tortorich, Vinnie with Dean Lorey. *Fitness Confidential.* Read by the author. Los Angeles: Pistachio Press, 2013. Audible audio ed., 7hr., 16min.

USDA National Agricultural Library, Food and Nutrition Information Center. "How Many Calories are in One Gram of Fat, Carbohydrate, or Protein?" Accessed October 22, 2020. *https:// www.nal.usda.gov/fnic/how-many-calories-are-one-gram-fat-carbohydrate-or-protein*

Volek, Jeff S., PhD, RD, and Stephen D. Phinney, MD, PhD. *The Art and Science of Low-Carbohydrate Performance.* New York: Beyond Obesity, LLC, 2012. Kindle.

CHAPTER 5

Centers for Disease Control and Prevention. "Seizure First Aid." last modified September 30, 2020. *https://www.cdc.gov/epilepsy/about/first-aid.htm*

Tortorich, Vinnie. "Fighting Seizures with Jim Abrahams and Susan Masino." November 25, 2016. In *Fitness Confidential Podcast.* Podcast, MP3 audio. *https://angriesttrainer.libsyn.com/podcast/fighting-seizures-with-jim-abrahams-and-susan-masino*

CHAPTER 6

Baxendale, Sallie. "Epilepsy on the Silver Screen in the 21st Century." *Epilepsy & Behavior* 57 pt. B (April 2016): 270-274. doi: 10.1016/j.yebeh.2015.12.044.

Eichenwald, Kurt. *A Mind Unraveled: A Memoir.* Read by the author. New York: Random House Audio, 2018. Audible audio ed., 14hr., 53 min.

Schneider, Joseph W. and Peter Conrad. "In the Closet with Illness: Epilepsy, Stigma Potential and Information Control." *Social Problems* 28 no. 1 (October 1980): 32–44. *https://doi.org/10.2307/800379*

Tian, Niu, MD, PhD, Michael Boring, MS, Rosemarie Kobau, MPH, Matthew M. Zack, MD, and Janet B. Croft, PhD. "Active Epilepsy and Seizure Control in Adults—United States, 2013 and 2015." *Morbidity and Mortality Weekly Report* 67 no 15 (April 20, 2018): 437–442. *http://dx.doi.org/10.15585/mmwr.mm6715a1external icon*

CHAPTER 7

Abrahams, Jim. "Mrs. Kelly." *Keto Lifestyle* (blog). The Charlie Foundation. Accessed October 22, 2020. *https://charliefoundation.org/mrs-kelly/*

"Drug Resistant Epilepsy and New AEDs: Two Perspectives." *Epilepsy Currents* 18 no. 5 (September-October, 2018): 304–306. doi:10.5698/1535-7597.18.5.304

Encyclopedia Britannica Online. s.v. "Hippocrates: Greek Physician." Accessed October 22, 2020. *https://www.britannica.com/biography/Hippocrates*

Epilepsy Foundation. "Phenytoin." Accessed October 22, 2020. *https://www.epilepsy.com/medications/phenytoin/advanced*

Greek Medicine.Net. "Fasting and Purification: The Physician Within." Accessed October 22, 2020. *http://www.greekmedicine.net/hygiene/Fasting_and_Purification.html*

"Fasting as Epilepsy Cure." *New York Times.* July 6, 1922.

Freeman, John M, MD. *Looking Back: A Career in Child Neurology.* Seattle: Book Surge Publishing. 2007.

Freeman, John M, MD, Millicent T. Kelly, RD, LD, Jennifer B. Freeman. *The Epilepsy Diet Treatment: An Introduction to the Ketogenic Diet.* New York: Demos, 1994.

Issu. "The Life of Raphael, by Giorgio Vasari, Introduced by Jill Burke—A Preview." Last modified April 5, 2016. *https://issuu. com/pallasatheneo/docs/raphael_issuu*

Janz,Deiter. "Epilepsy, Viewed Metaphysically: An Interpretation of the Biblical Story of the Epileptic Boy and of Raphael's Transfiguration." *Epilepsia* 27 (August 1986): 316–322. *https:// doi.org/10.1111/j.1528-1157.1986.tb03548.x*

Kossoff,Eric MD, Zahava Turner, RD, CSP, LDN, Sarah Doerrer, CPNP, Mackenzie Cervenka, MD, and Bobbie J. Henry, RD, LDN.*The Ketogenic and Modified Atkins Diets: Treatments for Epilepsy and Other Disorders*, 6th Edition. New York: Demos Health, 2016.

Lennox, William G. *Epilepsy and Related Disorders.* Little, Brown and Company, Boston, 1960. Vol 2: 734–739, 824–832.

Livingston, Samuel, MD. "Childhood Epilepsy: An Overview, 1936–1973." *Pediatric Annals* 2, no. 8 (August 1973): 10-22.

"Millicent Kelly and the Modern History of the Ketogenic Diet." The Charlie Foundation. April 24, 2018. YouTube Video, 8:47. *https://www.youtube.com/watch?v=Ma5t4ClKZSU*

MIT Internet Classics Archive. "On the Sacred Disease By Hippocrates." MIT Internet Classics Archive. Accessed October 22, 2020. *http://classics.mit.edu/Hippocrates/sacred.html*

Raphael Paintings. "The Transfiguration—by Raphael." Accessed October 22, 2020. *https://www.raphaelpaintings.org/the-transfiguration.jsp*

"Samuel Livingston Dies." *The Washington Post.* August 25, 1984.

US News and World Report Health, 2020 Best Diets Rankings. "Keto Diet: Expert Reviews." Accessed October 22, 2020. *https://health.usnews.com/best-diet/keto-diet/reviews*

Wheless, James W. "History and Origin of the Ketogenic Diet." In Epilepsy and the Ketogenic Diet, edited by Carl E. Stafstrom, MD, PhD and Jong M. Rho, MD, 31–38. Totowa, NJ: Humana Press, 2008.

Williams, Denis. "W. G. Lennox On Epilepsy." *Brain* 83 no. 4 (December 1960): 758–759. *https://doi.org/10.1093/brain/83.4.758*

Yagoda, Ben. "The True Story of Bernard Macfadden." *American Heritage.* December, 1981. *https://www.americanheritage.com/true-story-bernard-macfadden#2*

CHAPTER 8

Ede, Georgia. "Our Descent into Madness: Modern Diets and the Global Menal Health Crisis." Low Carb Down Under. April 21, 2018. YouTube video, 32:55. *https://www.youtube.com/watch?v=TXlVfwJ6RQU&t=184s*

Freeman, John M., MD. *Looking Back: A Career in Child Neurology.* Seattle: Book Surge Publishing. 2007.

Kossoff,Eric MD, Zahava Turner, RD, CSP, LDN, Sarah Doerrer, CPNP, Mackenzie Cervenka, MD, and Bobbie J. Henry, RD, LDN.*The Ketogenic and Modified Atkins Diets: Treatments for Epilepsy and Other Disorders*, 6th Edition. New York: Demos Health, 2016.

Swaminathan, Nikhil. "Why Does the Brain Need So Much Power?" *Scientific American.* April 29, 2008. *https://www.scientificamerican.com/article/why-does-the-brain-need-s/*

CHAPTER 9

Khullar, Dhruv, MD. "Doctors Getting 'Pimped.'" *Well* (blog). *The New York Times.* May 26, 2016. *https://well.blogs.nytimes.com/2016/05/26/doctors-getting-pimped/*

CHAPTER 10

EAT Forum. "The EAT-Lancet Commission on Food, Planet, Health." Accessed October 23, 2020. *https://eatforum.org/eat-lancet-commission/*

Kearns, Brad. "Vinnie Tortorich—Fitness Confidential Author, Celebrity Trainer." October 30, 2018. Get Over Yourself Podcast. MP3 audio, 1:14:57. *https://www.bradkearns.com/2018/10/30/vinnietortorich/#1537804290528-70f55232-6bc6*

Miko, Stephen. "The River, the Iceberg, and the Shit-detector." Criticism 33, no. 4 (1991): 503-25. *http://www.jstor.org/stable/23114990.*

Moodie, Alison. "Before You Read Another Health Study, Check Who's Funding the Research." *An Apple a Day* (blog). *The Guardian*, US Edition. December 12, 2016. *https://www.theguardian.com/lifeandstyle/2016/dec/12/studies-health-nutrition-sugar-coca-cola-marion-nestle*

Mountford, Sonia. "Why is Big Food in Bed with Dieticians? Follow the Money!" *BizNews.* May 30, 2015. *https://www.biznews.com/health/age-well/2015/05/30/why-is-big-food-in-bed-with-dietitians-follow-the-love-of-money*

Noakes, Tim and Markia Sboros. *Real Food On Trial: How the Diet Dictators Tried to Destroy a Top Scientist.* London: Columbus Publishing, 2019. Kindle.

Nutrition Coalition. "Who's On the Guidelines Committee." Updated March 6, 2019. *https://www.nutritioncoalition.us/ news/2020-dietary-guidelines-committee*

Nutrition Coalition. "Who We Are." Accessed October 22. 2020. *https://www.nutritioncoalition.us/about*

O'Brien, Robyn. "Widespread Panic and Coconuts: Follow the Money." *Robyn O'Brien* (blog). June 21, 2017. *https://robyno-brien.com/widespread-panic-coconuts-follow-money/*

Scher, Bret, MD. "Diet Doctor Podcast #21—Nina Teicholz." June 4, 2019. in *Diet Doctor Podcast.* Podcast. MP3 audio, 56:05. *https:// www.dietdoctor.com/diet-doctor-podcast-21-nina-teicholz*

Seymour, Colin. "Tim Noakes: 'If You've Got Lore of Running, Tear Out the Section on Nutrition.'" *Gone for a Run* (blog). February 2, 2012. *https://gonefora.run/tim-noakes-if-youve-got-lore-of-running-tear-out-the-section-on-nutrition*

Shahbandeh, M. "US Consumption of Edible Oils by Type 2019." Statista. January 30, 2020. *https://www.statista.com/statis-tics/301044/edible-oils-consumption-united-states-by-type/*

Teicholz, Nina. "Heart Breaker." *Gourmet,* June 2004. *http://www. gourmet.com.s3-website-us-east-1.amazonaws.com/maga-zine/2000s/2004/06/heart_breaker.html*

Teicholz, Nina. *The Big Fat Surprise: Why Butter, Meat, and Cheese Belong in a Healthy Diet.* New York: Simon and Schuster, 2014.

Torjensen, Ingrid. "WHO Pulls Support from Initiative Promoting Global Move to Plant Based Foods." *BMJ* 365 (April 9, 2019): 1700. *https://doi.org/10.1136/bmj.l1700*

University of Wisconsin—Madison. "What Determines Sky's Colors At Sunrise And Sunset?." ScienceDaily. Accessed October 22, 2020. *www.sciencedaily.com/releases/2007/11/071108135522. htm* ().

CHAPTER 11

Lenzkes, Brian and Tro Kalayjian. "Episode 26: Seizure Salad." April 3, 2019. in *Low Carb MD Podcast.* Podcast, MP3 audio. 50:20. *https://lowcarbmd.com/size/5/?search=seizure+salad*

CHAPTER 12

Glatter, MD, Robert. "The Price to Pay for Eating Highly Processed Carbohydrates." *Forbes.* June 30, 2013. *https://www.forbes.com/ sites/robertglatter/2013/06/30/the-price-to-pay-for-eating-highly-processed-carbohydrates/#7c4a5c734f1d*

Harcombe, Zoë, PhD. "Carbohydrate Addiction—Part 1 With Dr. Robert Cywes." *Diet & Health Today.* June 6, 2018. Produced by Zoë Harcombe. Podcast, MP3 audio. 34:14. *https://podcasts. apple.com/us/podcast/diet-and-health-today/id439578113*

The JAMA Network Journals. "Long-term followup of type of bariatric surgery finds regain of weight, decrease in diabetes remission." ScienceDaily. August 5, 2015. *www.sciencedaily. com/releases/2015/08/150805121833.htm*

Vocino, Anna. *Eat Happy: Gluten Free, Grain Free, Low Carb Recipes for a Joyful Life.* Los Angeles: Telemachus Press, 2016.

Vocino, Anna. "My Story." Anna Vocino, Eat Happy. Accessed October 23, 2020. *https://annavocino.com/my-story/*

Ye, Fang, Xiao-Jia Li, Wan-Lin Jiang , Hong-Bin Sun, and Jie Liu. "Efficacy of and patient compliance with a ketogenic diet in adults with intractable epilepsy: a meta-analysis." *Journal of*

Clinical Neurology 11 no. 1 (January 2015): 26-31. *https://pubmed. ncbi.nlm.nih.gov/25628734/*

CHAPTER 13
Ketonix Breath Ketone Analyzer. "Advantages Using Ketonix." Accessed October 25, 2020 *https://www.ketonix.com/keto- nix-advantage*

CHAPTER 14
Clear, James. *Atomic Habits: An Easy & Proven Way to Build Good Habits & Break Bad Ones*. Read by the author. New York: Pen- guin Audio, 2018. Audible audio ed., 5hrs, 25 min.

Cywes, Robert. "Arrogant Integrity." Facebook video. February 19, 2020. *https://www.facebook.com/carbaddictiondoc/vid- eos/186764202547709/*

Hite, Adele, PhD, MPH, RDN. "American Diabetes Association endorses low-carb diet as option." Diet Doctor, April 25, 2019. *https://www.dietdoctor.com/american-diabetes-association-en- dorses-low-carb-diet-as-option*

McGonigal, Kelly, PhD. *The Willpower Instinct: How Self-Control Works, Why it Matters, and What You Can Do to Get More of It*. New York: Avery, 2012.

CHAPTER 15
Moore, Jimmy. "1359: Jade Nelson Finds The Train Inside Of Her With Keto Epilepsy Journey." January 30, 2018. In *The Livin' La Vida Low Carb Show*. Produced by Jimmy Moore. Podcast, MP3 audio, 40:07. *https://livinlavidalowcarb.com/ llvlc-pod/2018/01/30/1359-jade-nelson-finds-the-train-inside- of-her-with-keto-epilepsy-journey/*

Nelson, Jade. "Epilepsy & Keto: My Journey of Healing in the Kitchen." Keto Con 2018. July 16, 2018. YouTube Video, 37:45. *https://www.youtube.com/watch?v=IjzXSEVK2do*

Nelson, Jade. "Meet Jade." Jade Nelson: Hope, Strength, and Wisdom. Accessed October 23, 2020. *https://www.jadenelson.net*

CHAPTER 16

Cunnane, Stephen C, and Michael A Crawford. "Survival Of The Fattest: Fat Babies Were The Key To Evolution Of The Large Human Brain." *Comparative Biochemistry and Physiology. Part A, Molecular & Integrative Physiology* 136, no. 1 (September 2003): 17–26. doi:10.1016/s1095-6433(03)00048-5

Kent, Chelsea, Shannon L. Kesl, PhD, Stacy A. Hodges, DVM, Loren Nations, DVM, DABVP. "Ketopet Sanctuary: Ketosis, Cancer And Canines—Part 2." *Innovative Veterinary Care.* June 25, 2019. *https://ivcjournal.com/ketopet-sanctuary-keto-sis-cancer-part-2/*

KetoPet, About Us."Our Beginning: A Keto Sanctuary for Dogs with Cancer." Accessed October 23, 2020. *https://www.ketop-etsanctuary.com/pages/about-us*

Kunkle, Frederick. "Alzheimer's Spurs the Fearful to Change Their Lives to Delay It." *Washington Post.* July 4, 2015. *https://www.washingtonpost.com/local/social-issues/fear-of-alzheimers-is-everywhere-but-its-spurring-some-people-to-change-their-lives-for-the-better/2015/07/04/c0600046-192a-11e5-93b7-5eddc056ad8a_story.html*

Masino, Susan, M Kawamura, Jr, D. Wasser, L.T Pomeroy, and D.N Ruskin. "Adenosine, Ketogenic Diet and Epilepsy: the Emerging Therapeutic Relationship Between Metabolism and Brain Activity." *Current Neuropharmacology* 7, no. 3 (March 2009): 257–68. doi:10.2174/157015909789152164

Newport, Mary, MD. "Improvement with MCTs and Ketone Monoester in a Case of Alzheimer's: What Happened and Why?" PowerPoint presentation at Metabolic Health Summit, Long Beach CA, January 30–February 2, 2020. *https://metabolichealthsummit.com/products/mhs-2020-video-presentations-panels-special-interest-forums-package*

Nobel Media AB 2020. "Francis Crick—Facts." Nobel Prize. Accessed October 23, 2020. *https://www.nobelprize.org/prizes/medicine/1962/crick/facts/*

Nobel Media AB 2020. "Otto Warburg—Facts," Nobel Prize. Accessed October 23, 2020. *https://www.nobelprize.org/prizes/medicine/1931/warburg/facts/*

PetMD. "Anal Gland Cancer in Dogs." July 2, 2008. Accessed October 23, 2020. *https://www.petmd.com/dog/conditions/cancer/c_multi_adenocarcinoma_anal*

Rho, John, MD. "Diet and the Brain: Is there a Bona Fide Scientific Connection?" PowerPoint presentation, Metabolic Health Summit, Long Beach CA, January 30, 2020. *https://metabolichealthsummit.com/products/mhs-2020-video-presentations-panels-special-interest-forums-package*

Seyfried, Thomas N, George Yu, Joseph C. Maroon, and Dominic P. D'Agostino. "Press-pulse: a novel therapeutic strategy for the metabolic management of cancer." *Nutrition & metabolism* 14 no. 19. February 23, 2017). doi:10.1186/s12986-017-0178-2

Seyfried, Thomas N., Laura Shelton, Gabriel Arismendi-Morillo, Miriam Kalamian, Ahmed Elsakka, Joseph Maroon, and Purna Mukherjee. "Provocative Question: Should Ketogenic Metabolic Therapy Become the Standard of Care for Glioblastoma?" *Neurochemical Research* 44 (October 2019): 2392–2404. *https://doi.org/10.1007/s11064-019-02795-4*

US National Library of Medicine, National Institutes of Health. "Search of: Ketogenic." PubMed. Accessed October 26, 2020. *https://pubmed.ncbi.nlm.nih.gov/?term=ketogenic*

US National Library of Medicine, National Institutes of Health. "Search of: Ketogenic." ClinicalTrials.gov. Accessed October 23, 2020. *https://clinicaltrials.gov/ct2/results?term=ketogenic&-Search=Apply&recrs=b&recrs=a&recrs=f&recrs=d&recrs=e&recrs=m&age_v=&gndr=&type=&rslt*

Zupec-Kania, Beth. "Thomas Seyfried, PhD, Professor, Researcher And Pioneer Of Cancer As A Metabolic Disease." *Keto Lifestyle* (blog). The Charlie Foundation for Ketogenic Therapies. Accessed October 23, 2020. *https://charliefoundation.org/dr-seyfried-discusses-ketogenic-diet/*

CHAPTER 17

American Association of Family Physicians. "All Policies: Primary Care" Accessed October 23, 2020. *https://www.aafp.org/about/policies/all/primary-care.html*

Bocchicchio, Ben, PhD. "The Power Of The Muscle System In The Management Of Metabolic Dysfunction." PowerPoint presentation. Low Carb USA Virtual San Diego 2020 Conference, August 28, 2020. *https://www.lowcarbusa.org/videos/premium-event-videos/virtual-san-diego-2020-livestream/*

BrainyQuote. "Zig Ziglar Quotes." Accessed October 23, 2020. *https://www.brainyquote.com/quotes/zig_ziglar_387369*

Cornell, Chris S. "Online Group Coaching Aims to Help Participants Maintain Benefits of Low Carb & Fasting; Manage Stress During These Difficult Times." Doctor Tro's Medical Weight Loss and Direct Primare Care. April 30, 2020. *https://www.doctortro.com/online-town-hall-meeting-aims-to-help-partic-*

ipants-maintain-benefits-of-low-carb-manage-stress-during-
these-difficult-times/

Lenzkes, Brian, MD. "Physician Burnout: The Silent Epidemic in
Healthcare." PowerPoint presentation. Low Carb USA Virtual San Diego 2020 Conference, August 27, 2020. *https://www.
lowcarbusa.org/videos/premium-event-videos/virtual-san-di-
ego-2020-livestream/*

Lenzkes, Brian MD and Tro Kalayjian, MD. "Episode 109: Dr. Kristin Baier." May 27, 2020. In *Low Carb MD Podcast*. Podcast,
MP3 audio. 47:02. *https://lowcarbmd.com/episode-109-dr-kris-
tin-baier*

Norbeck, Timothy B. "Drivers Of Health Care Costs. A Physicians
Foundation White Paper—Second Of A Three-Part Series."
Missouri Medicine 110, no. 2 (March–April 2013): 113–8. *https://
www.ncbi.nlm.nih.gov/pmc/articles/PMC6179664/*

Sanders, Brian and Brian Lenzkes. "The Future of Medicine, Aligning Incentives, and Fixing the Broken Healthcare (Sickcare)
System." June 23, 2020, in *Peak Human*. Podcast, MP3 audio,
1:20:14. *https://www.peak-human.com/post/the-future-of-medi-
cine-aligning-incentives-and-fixing-the-broken-healthcare-sick-
care-system*

Scher, Bret, MD. "Diet Doctor Podcast #41–Brian Lenzkes." March
11, 2020, on *Diet Doctor Podcast*. Podcast, MP3 audio, 54:25.
*https://www.dietdoctor.com/diet-doctor-podcast-41-brian-lenz-
kes*

Ye, Fang, Xiao-Jia Li, Wan-Lin Jiang , Hong-Bin Sun, and Jie Liu.
"Efficacy of and Patient Compliance With a Ketogenic Diet in
Adults With Intractable Epilepsy: A Meta-Analysis." *Journal of
Clinical Neurology* 11 no. 1 (January 2015): 26–31. *https://pubmed.
ncbi.nlm.nih.gov/25628734/*

AFTERWORD

Centers for Disease Control and Prevention. "Seizure First Aid." Last modified September 30, 2020. *https://www.cdc.gov/epilepsy/about/first-aid.htm*

Jeong, Ken. *You Complete Me, Ho.* Netflix Special. 2019.

Printed in Great Britain
by Amazon

11511112R00153